国際論文 English 投稿ハンドブック
カバーレター作成・査読コメントへの返答

C.S.Langham（日本大学特任教授）著

COMMUNICATION WITH EDITORS AND REVIEWERS: A GUIDE TO COVER LETTERS, RESEARCH HIGHLIGHTS, RESPONDING TO REVIEWERS' COMMENTS, COMMON ERRORS AND FREQUENTLY USED WORDS

医歯薬出版株式会社

This book is originally published in Japanese
under the title of :

Kokusai Ronbun Ingurisshu Toko Handobukku
(Communication with editors and reviewers)

C. S. Langham
　　Professor at Nihon University School of Dentistry

ⓒ 2017　1st ed.

ISHIYAKU PUBLISHERS, INC.
　7-10, Honkomagome 1 chome, Bunkyo-ku,
　Tokyo 113-8612, Japan

Introduction

Over a period of 30 years in Japan, I have provided editorial assistance to colleagues writing research papers in English. Although I currently get fewer requests for help, the number of authors requiring assistance with issues connected with the submission process and communication with editors and reviewers has increased. This book is intended to help authors with problems that arise after the manuscript has been completed, and deals with cover letters for initial submissions and revised manuscripts, research highlights, and replies to reviewers' comments. It introduces common errors and has a section on frequently used words. Examples are applicable to different fields and are not specific to a particular genre.

Acknowledgments

Thanks are due to my colleagues at the Journal of Oral science, particularly Professor N. Koshikawa, Editor in Chief, who has shown an interest in this work and provided useful examples of reviewers' comments and authors' responses. I am indebted to Dr. Noriko Yamaguchi of the Institute of Agro-environmental Sciences for allowing access to correspondence and examples of communication with editors and reviewers. I also wish to acknowledge my colleague and friend, Brian Purdue of Tsukuba University, with whom I have had many valuable discussions concerning academic and scientific English discourse. Finally, I wish to acknowledge participants in the English language skills programs at the National Institute of Advanced Industrial Science and Technology, and Tsukuba Center for Institutes, who have asked questions about responding to reviewers' comments and, in doing so, contributed to this book. To all of these people, I am extremely grateful.

Clive Langham
Nihon University
School of Dentistry
Ochanomizu, Tokyo
December 1st, 2016

CONTENTS

Introduction
Acknowledgments

Part 1 Cover letters for initial submissions 1

   1 Cover letter 1 (Title, names of authors, declarations, corresponding author's contact details) 2
   2 Cover letter 2 (Research highlights: topic, methods, findings) 10
   3 Cover letter 3 (Research highlights: topic, importance of the paper, target audience) 16
   4 Cover letter 4 (Research highlights in 5 steps) 22
   5 Cover letter 5 (How to answer questions listed in the Instructions to Authors) 30

  ● 論文の初回投稿時に使用するカバーレター（原稿送り状）の書き方を解説します。

Part 2 Cover letters for submission of revised manuscripts 41

   1 Basic cover letter with no explanation of responses to reviewers' comments 42
   2 Cover letter that includes a brief description of the main changes to the manuscript 44
   3 Cover letter including detailed explanations of the main changes to the manuscript (1) 52
   4 Cover letter including detailed explanations of the main changes to the manuscript (2) 62

  ● 査読者の指摘に従って論文を修正した後、修正原稿を再投稿する際に使用するカバーレターの書き方を解説します。

Part 3 Research highlights 69

   1 Example of detailed research highlights 70
   2 Analysis of the main functions 71
   3 Analysis of sentences, expressions and vocabulary 72

  ● 論文投稿時のカバーレターには，研究の背景・手法・結果などをまとめた「研究ハイライト」を含めることがよくあります。この章では，「研究ハイライト」の構成と書き方を説明します。

Part 4 How to handle questions concerning research highlights ... 79

   1 Subject, topic, context, background 80
   2 Research gap/originality 84
   3 Importance of the work 86
   4 Impact on the field 88
   5 Fit to the journal 90

  ● 雑誌の投稿規定の中には，「研究ハイライト」に含めるべき事項について質問形式で問われていることがあります。この章では，よくある質問事項に対する説明文の例を紹介します。

Part 5 Responding to reviewers' comments 93
1 Simple revisions 94
2 Comments concerning language 100
3 Requests for more information 102
4 Clarifying a point 108
5 Explaining why you cannot comply with a reviewer's request 112
6 Explaining why you do not want to make a suggested change 118
7 Responding to critical comments 125

● 査読者からの指摘にどのように対応するか，修正内容をどのように説明するか，査読者の提案に応じられない場合はどうすればよいか…など，査読コメントへの返答文を執筆する際の注意事項を解説します。

Part 6 Common errors 131
1 Grammar 132
2 Vocabulary 150
3 Expressions 158

● 査読コメントへの対応時に日本人が犯しがちな文法・単語・表現に関する間違いと，正しい文章に直すためのアドバイスをまとめました。

Part 7 Index of frequently used words 165

● 査読コメントに返答する際によく用いる単語とその用例をまとめました。

Notes on responding to reviewers' comments
1 Which word should I use, 'enclosed' or 'attached'? 15
2 Is extremely formal language appropriate in communication with editors and reviewers? 21
3 Thanking reviewers 28
4 Words with the prefix re 39
5 How do you handle a reviewer's comment that is unclear? 50
6 How long does it take to revise and resubmit a paper? 54
7 Comments concerning the quality of English 61
8 Apologizing 92
9 How short can responses to reviewers' comments be? 98
10 Grammar choices: We have added vs We added 117
11 Don't get mad, get formal 173

● 査読コメントへの返答時の注意事項や関連する話題などを11のコラムにまとめました。

Part 1
Cover letters for initial submissions

With online submissions becoming common, the need for a cover letter is changing. A lot depends on the discipline. In humanities, for example, cover letters are not considered essential. In social sciences, they are more common, but consist only of a brief statement of basic information about the contents of the paper. In life science subjects, the need is greater and letters are longer with more detailed information. In biomedicine, there is a lot of competition for journal space, and a well-written cover letter can influence the outcome of the submission. Cover letters can be an important part of the submission process, and the ability to write one an essential skill. In part 1, I provide five examples each followed by a Quick Guide that explains the contents and focuses on useful words, phrases and sentences.

Cover letter 1

This letter contains the following information: **title of the manuscript, names of the authors, a declaration stating the manuscript has not been published or submitted elsewhere** and **the corresponding author's contact details.**

Note

In each of the cover letters 1 to 5, section headings are shown in blue. These are for the purposes of explanation only. Also in this letter only, I show how to write the editor's name and address at the top of the letter, and the corresponding author's contact details at the bottom.

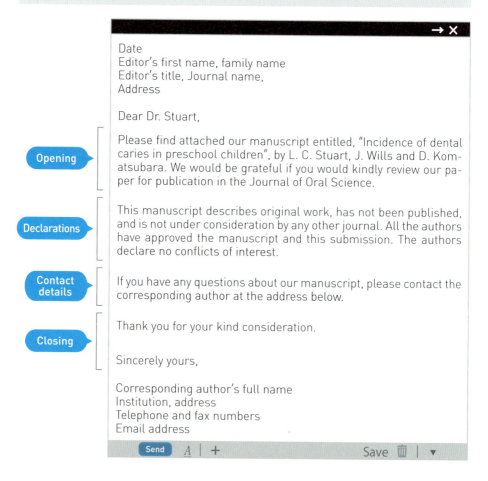

Part 1 Cover letters for initial submissions

Key sentences

Here is the same letter with the key sentences numbered. Each numbered sentence appears in the Quick Guide on page 4 with an explanation and further examples.

1. **Please find attached our manuscript entitled**, "Incidence of dental caries in preschool children", **by** L. C. Stuart, J. Wills and D. Komatsubara.

2. We would be grateful if you would kindly review our paper for publication in (name of the journal).

3. This manuscript describes original work, has not been published, and is not under consideration by any other journal.

4. All the authors have approved the manuscript and this submission.

5. The authors declare no conflicts of interest.

6. If you have any questions about our manuscript, please contact the corresponding author at the address given below.

7. Thank you for your kind consideration.

8. Sincerely yours,

Quick Guide 1 »»»

Here the key sentences from cover letter 1 are explained and further examples given.

1. The opening sentence　書き出し

- <u>Please find attached our manuscript entitled</u>, "Incidence of dental caries in pre-school children", **by** L. C. Stuart, J. Wills and D. Komatsubara.

Explanation

The opening sentence gives the title of the paper and the names of the authors. The verb **attached** is used in the phrase, **Please find attached our manuscript entitled**, (title of paper). When stating the title of the manuscript, it is possible to use **entitled** or **titled**. The word entitled is more frequently used than titled.

Examples

- <u>Attached please find our manuscript entitled</u>, "Incidence of dental caries in preschool children", <u>which we are submitting for consideration for publication in</u> (name of the journal).
- <u>We are pleased to submit our manuscript entitled</u>, "Incidence of dental caries in preschool children" <u>for publication in</u> (name of the journal).
- <u>We wish to submit our paper entitled</u>, "Incidence of dental caries in preschool children" by L. C. Stuart, J. Wills and D. Komatsubara.
- <u>Attached is a paper entitled</u>, "Incidence of dental caries in preschool children" by J. Ogata, L. C. Stuart and T. J. Williams.
- <u>I am writing to submit our manuscript entitled</u>, "Incidence of dental caries in preschool children", <u>for consideration for publication in</u> (name of the journal).
- <u>We are submitting our paper entitled</u>, "Incidence of dental caries in pre-school children in Japan" <u>for publication in</u> (name of the journal).
- <u>We would like to submit our paper entitled</u>, "Incidence of dental caries in pre-school children in Japan" <u>for publication in</u> (name of the journal).

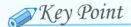 *Key Point*

● 論文投稿時のカバーレターでは，はじめに 'Please find attached our manuscript entitled, (論文のタイトル)' などの表現を用いて論文のタイトルを示す．

2. Asking for the paper to be reviewed　査読の依頼

- <u>We would be grateful if you would kindly review our paper for publication in</u> (name of the journal).

Explanation

The authors request that their paper is reviewed using the polite expression:
We would be grateful if you would kindly review our paper for publication in (name of the journal).

Examples

- <u>We wish to have our manuscript considered for publication in</u> (name of the journal).
- <u>We would like to have the manuscript considered for publication in</u> (name of the journal).
- <u>We would be most grateful if you would kindly review our manuscript</u>.
- <u>We would be grateful if you would consider our paper for publication in</u> (name of the journal).

Key Point

● 続いて，添付した論文の査読を依頼する．
● 依頼の際は，'We would be grateful' 'We would like to' などの丁寧な表現を用いるとよい．

3. Statement that the paper has never been published　二重投稿ではないことの誓約

- <u>This manuscript describes original work, has not been published, and is not under consideration by any other journal</u>.

1.1 Cover letter 1　　5

Explanation

The authors make three declarations: 1) the work is original 2) it has not been published 3) it has not been submitted elsewhere.

Examples

- <u>We confirm that the manuscript is completely our own work, has not been published, and is not under consideration for publication elsewhere.</u>
- <u>This work is original. The contents have not been accepted by any other journal, and the paper has not been submitted elsewhere.</u>
- <u>The work described here has not been published before, has not been submitted for publication to any other journals, and will not be published elsewhere while under review at</u> (name of the journal).
- <u>This paper has not been published, is not currently submitted for publication elsewhere, nor will be submitted elsewhere while under review at</u> (name of the journal).
- <u>None of the work described in this paper has been published before, and is not currently being submitted to another journal.</u>
- <u>This paper has not been published before, and is not under consideration by another journal.</u>

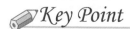Key Point

● 論文が二重投稿ではないことを必ず示す。

---

4. Statement that all the authors have approved the manuscript and this submission
共著者全員が原稿の内容と投稿に同意していることの誓約

- <u>All the authors have approved the manuscript and this submission.</u>

Explanation

It is essential to state that the authors have all approved the submission of the paper. Please note that this example uses the words, **the manuscript and this submission.**

Examples

- **All of the authors have seen the final version of this manuscript and agreed to its submission**.
- **All the authors have approved the submission of this paper to**（name of the journal）.
- **All the authors have agreed the submission of this paper to**（name of the journal）.

🖍 Key Point

● 共著者全員が原稿の内容と雑誌への投稿に同意していることを必ず示す．

[5. Statement that there are no conflicts of interest
利益相反がないことの誓約]

- **The authors declare no conflicts of interest**.

Explanation

It is necessary to state that there are no conflicts of interest.

Examples

- **There are no conflicts of interest**.
- **We have no conflicts of interest to report**.
- **There are no conflicts of interest to disclose**.

🖍 Key Point

● 利益相反（conflict of interest: COI）がないことを必ず示す．

[6. The corresponding author's contact details are given
責任著者の連絡先]

- **If you have any questions about our manuscript, please contact the corresponding author at the address given below**.

Explanation

It is important to give the corresponding author's contact details.

Examples

- Questions concerning this manuscript should be addressed to the corresponding author at the following address.
- Any correspondence should be directed to me at the following address.
- If you require any more information, please contact the corresponding author at the address below.
- Should you require any more information about our manuscript, please contact the corresponding author at the address given below.

Key Point

● 責任著者（corresponding author, 連絡著者ともよばれる）の連絡先を必ず明記する.

7. Thanking the editor　編集者への感謝

- Thank you for your kind consideration.

Explanation

The authors express their thanks to the editor.

Examples

- Thank you for your attention.
- Thank you for considering our manuscript.
- Thank you very much for your consideration.
- Thank you in advance for your cooperation.
- We very much appreciate your consideration.
- Thank you for considering our manuscript for review. We appreciate your time and look forward to hearing from you in due course.

Key Point

● 日本語の「よろしくお願いします」の代わりに，英語では 'Thank you for your kind consideration.' などの表現を用いる.

8. Finishing the letter　結びの挨拶

- **Sincerely yours**,

Explanation

The authors close the letter with the expression, **Sincerely yours**.

Examples

- **Kind regards**,
- **Sincerely**,
- **Yours sincerely**,
- **Respectfully yours**,

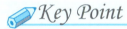

Key Point

- カバーレターの結びには 'Sincerely yours,' などを用いる.

Cover letter 2

This letter includes a **paragraph on research highlights***, which is divided into **topic**, **methods** and **findings**.

*Note on research highlights

Most publishers of scientific journals request that authors include four or five lines of research highlights on the first page of their article in a position just above the abstract. This is to help readers understand the contents quickly and easily, and to aid tracking by Internet search engines.
Research highlights are also used in cover letters for initial submissions and resubmitted papers, and are particularly useful because they allow editors to quickly understand the main points of the research and make a speedy decision about the review process.

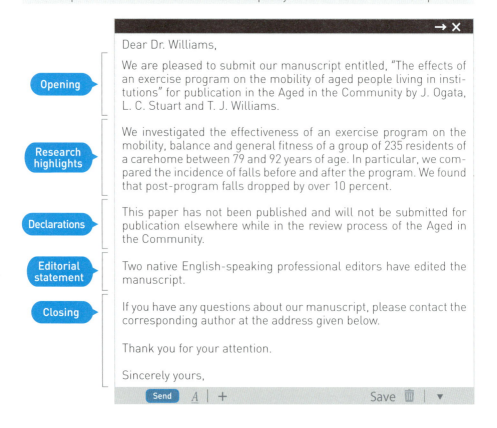

Opening

Dear Dr. Williams,

We are pleased to submit our manuscript entitled, "The effects of an exercise program on the mobility of aged people living in institutions" for publication in the Aged in the Community by J. Ogata, L. C. Stuart and T. J. Williams.

Research highlights

We investigated the effectiveness of an exercise program on the mobility, balance and general fitness of a group of 235 residents of a carehome between 79 and 92 years of age. In particular, we compared the incidence of falls before and after the program. We found that post-program falls dropped by over 10 percent.

Declarations

This paper has not been published and will not be submitted for publication elsewhere while in the review process of the Aged in the Community.

Editorial statement

Two native English-speaking professional editors have edited the manuscript.

Closing

If you have any questions about our manuscript, please contact the corresponding author at the address given below.

Thank you for your attention.

Sincerely yours,

Key sentences

Here is the same letter with the key sentences numbered. Each numbered sentence appears in the Quick Guide on page 12 with an explanation and further examples.

1. <u>**We investigated** the effectiveness of an exercise program on the mobility, balance and general fitness of a group of 235 residents of a carehome between 79 and 92 years of age.</u>

2. <u>**In particular, we compared** the incidence of falls before and after the program.</u>

3. <u>**We found that** post-program falls dropped by over 10 percent.</u>

4. <u>**This paper has not been published and will not be submitted for publication elsewhere while in the review process of** (name of the journal).</u>

5. <u>**Two native English-speaking professional editors have edited the manuscript.**</u>

Quick Guide 2 »»»

In this quick guide, the key sentences from cover letter 2 are explained and further examples given.

> **1. State the research topic without repeating the title of the paper** 論文のタイトルとは表現を変えて研究テーマを述べる

- **We investigated** the effectiveness of an exercise program on the mobility, balance and general fitness of a group of 235 residents of a carehome between 79 and 92 years of age.

Explanation

The authors use the word **investigated** to introduce the main research theme. The following verbs could also be used: **assessed, evaluated, focused on, looked at, measured, studied.**

Examples

- **We focused on/studied** the effectiveness of an exercise program.
- **We looked at/evaluated** the effectiveness of an exercise program.

🖉 Key Point

● 研究テーマを紹介するときは 'investigated' 'focused on' 'looked at' などを用いる。

> **2. Introduce the methods** 方法を紹介する

- **In particular, we compared** the incidence of falls before and after the program.

Explanation

The authors focus on what was done. Commonly used verbs are: **analyzed, assessed, compared, measured.**

Examples

- **We assessed** the effects of the exercise program on mobility.
- **We measured** the incidence and severity of falls before and after the exercise program.

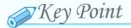*Key Point*

● 研究の方法について述べるときは 'analyzed' 'assessed' 'measured' などを用いる.

3. Introduce the main findings　主な結果を紹介する

- **We found that** post-program falls dropped by over 10 percent.

Explanation

The word **found** is used to introduce the results. Please note that if you have several different findings to report, it is possible to repeat the word **found** using the following expression, **it was also found**, in the same paragraph without worrying about repetition. This could be followed by the expression, **Another thing we found was that**（+ result）.

Examples

- **We found that** falls decreased/went down/dropped by over 10 percent.
- **We also found that** mobility improved.
- **Another thing we found was that** fewer patients were confined to their beds.
- **Our results show that** fewer patients were confined to their beds.

Key Point

● 研究結果については，'We found that' に続けて主な結果を説明する.
● 複数の結果について触れるときは，'It was also found' や 'Another thing we found was that' などを用いるとよい.

4. Declaration that the paper has not been published elsewhere　二重投稿ではないことを誓約する

- **This paper has not been published and will not be submitted for publication elsewhere while in the review process of**（name of the journal）.

Explanation

It is necessary to state that the paper has not been published elsewhere.

Examples

- This manuscript has not been published and is not under review elsewhere.
- We certify that this submission has not been published and is not under review at any other journal.

5. Statement concerning proof of editing
英文校正を受けたことを述べる

- Two native English-speaking professional editors have edited the manuscript.

Explanation

Many authors, for whom English is not their first language, have their papers checked by editing companies. If you do this, it is a good idea to provide a statement that the paper has been professionally edited.

Examples

- Our paper has been professionally edited by two native-English speakers.
- This paper has been professionally edited.
- Our paper has been edited by a native speaker of English, who is familiar with scientific English.
- A certificate from an editing company is attached stating that the manuscript has been professionally edited.
- The manuscript has been edited by two professional editors.

If your paper has been edited by a proofreading company and you have a certificate to prove it, these sentences can be used.

- Certification is attached.
- Proof of professional editing is attached.

🖉 Key Point

- 英文校正（英文校閲）を受けた場合は，そのことを明記するとよい．
- 英文校正業者による証明書を添付する場合は，'Certification is attached.' と説明する．

Notes on responding to reviewers' comments

1

Which word should I use, 'enclosed' or 'attached'?

'enclosed'? 'attached'? どちらを使うべきか？

The word 'enclose' means to put something inside an envelope in addition to a letter. It is commonly used in business letters where other documents are also being sent in an envelope. Here is an example:
- *Please find enclosed an agenda for the meeting.*

The word enclosed can only be used in an email if the information you are sending is contained within the text of the email itself. Here is an example:
- *You will find enclosed at the bottom of this email a list of the items we wish to order.*

<u>Attached</u> is used when you are sending a separate document containing information or data with your email. Here are some examples.
- *Please find attached a copy of our manuscript.*
- *We are attaching a revised version of our manuscript.*
- *We have attached our point-to-point responses to the reviewers' comments.*

Cover letter 3

This letter has a short paragraph on research highlights in which the following information is stated: **topic, importance of the paper, target audience**.

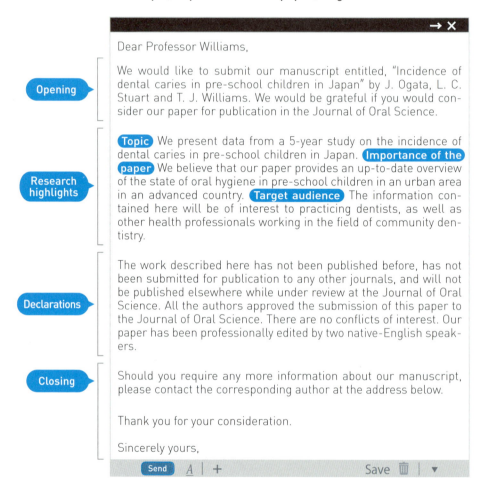

Key sentences

Here is the same letter with the key sentences numbered. Each numbered sentence appears in the Quick Guide on page 18 with an explanation and further examples.

1. **We present** data from a 5-year study on the incidence of dental caries in pre-school children in Japan.

2. **We believe that our paper provides** an up-to-date overview of the state of oral hygiene in pre-school children in an urban area in an advanced country.

3. **The information contained here will be of interest to** practicing dentists, as well as other health professionals working in the field of community dentistry.

Quick Guide 3 »»

In this quick guide, the key sentences from cover letter 3 are explained and further examples given.

> **1. Start the paragraph on research highlights by stating the topic without repeating the title** 研究ハイライトの書き出し—論文のタイトルとは表現を変えて研究のトピックを紹介する

- <u>We present</u> data from a 5-year study on the incidence of dental caries in pre-school children in Japan.

Explanation

This is the opening sentence of the paragraph on research highlights. The authors briefly explain the topic of the paper, but do not repeat the title itself. As shown in the examples below, the verbs **focus on, introduce, look at** and **report** are commonly used when introducing the research theme.

Examples

Here are ways of introducing the topic using **focus on, introduce, look at, report**.

- <u>We focus on</u> data from a 5-year study of the incidence of dental caries in pre-school children in Japan.
- <u>We introduce</u> data from a 5-year study of the incidence of dental caries in pre-school children in Japan.
- <u>We look at</u> data from a 5-year study of the incidence of dental caries in pre-school children in Japan.
- <u>We report</u> data from a 5-year study of the incidence of dental caries in pre-school children in Japan.

✏ Key Point

● 研究ハイライト（research highlights）の書き出しは，'investigate' 'focus on' 'look at' などの動詞を用いて研究テーマを簡潔に紹介する．

2. The authors state the importance of the paper
論文の重要性について述べる

- **We believe that our paper provides** an up-to-date overview of the state of oral hygiene in pre-school children in an urban area in an advanced country.

Explanation

The authors state the importance of their paper using the verb, **believe**. It is also possible to use **think** and **consider**.

Examples

- **We think that these results are important in terms of** oral hygiene in pre-school children in an urban area in an advanced country.
- **We think that these findings will add to existing knowledge of** oral hygiene in pre-school children in an urban area in an advanced country.
- **We consider that the results reported here are important in terms of** oral hygiene in pre-school children in an urban area in an advanced country.
- **We consider that our observations will add to the understanding of** oral hygiene in pre-school children in an urban area in an advanced country.
- **We believe that the reported data will contribute to understanding of** oral hygiene in pre-school children in an urban area in an advanced country.
- **These results are important in terms of** our understanding of the state of oral hygiene in pre-school children in an urban area in an advanced country.

Please note the following grammar patterns for the word **understanding**. The patterns are slightly different but the meaning is the same.

- We believe that the reported data will **contribute to understanding of** the state of oral hygiene in pre-school children in an urban area in an advanced country.
- We believe that the reported data will **contribute to our understanding of** the state of oral hygiene in pre-school children in an urban area in an advanced country.
- We believe that the reported data will **contribute to the understanding of** the state of oral hygiene in pre-school children in an urban area in an advanced country.

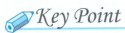Key Point

- 論文の重要性について 'believe' 'think' 'consider' などを用いてアピールする。

3. The authors refer to the target audience
ターゲットとする読者層を説明する

- <u>The information contained here will be of interest to</u> practicing dentists, as well as other health professionals working in the field of community dentistry.

Explanation

It is important to mention the target audience. The phrase, **will be of interest to**, is used. At the beginning of the sentence, you can use the following nouns: **data, findings, information, results**. The following verbs can be used: **contained, described, presented, reported**.

Here is an example.

- The (<u>data</u>, <u>findings</u>, <u>information</u>, <u>results</u>) (<u>contained</u>, <u>described</u>, <u>presented</u>, <u>reported</u>) (<u>here/in this paper</u>) will be of interest to (<u>dental hygienists</u>, <u>practicing dentists</u>, <u>people in the field of community dentistry</u>, <u>researchers working on</u> + topic).

Examples

- <u>The results reported here will be of interest to those working in</u> community dentistry.
- <u>We think the data reported in this paper will be of interest to those working in</u> community dentistry.
- <u>We consider that these findings will be of interest to researchers working on</u> oral hygiene.
- <u>We consider that these findings will be of interest to researchers working in the field of</u> community dentistry.
- <u>We believe the results are of interest to readers of</u> (name of the journal).

✏️ Key Point

- この論文がどのような読者層をターゲットとしているかを説明する。
- X（論文の内容）がY（読者層）にとって魅力的であることを示すためには、'X will be of interest to Y' を用いるとよい。

Notes on responding to reviewers' comments

2

Is extremely formal language appropriate in communication with editors and reviewers?

編集者・査読者とのやりとりで，過度に格式ばった表現は適切か？

Written communication with editors and reviewers should be formal as the context is a professional one and you are not usually acquainted with the person you are replying to. There is, however, a danger of being too formal and using words and sentences that are not appropriate for the situation. Below you will find two examples where the language used is very formal.

1-1. We are submitting <u>herewith</u> our manuscript entitled, (title of paper).
1-2. We are submitting our manuscript entitled, (title of paper).

In example 1-1, the word <u>herewith</u> is very formal and generally used in legal documents. For these reasons, it has been deleted.

2-1. Please find <u>appended</u> our responses to the reviewers' comments.
2-2. Please find attached our responses to the reviewers' comments.

In example 2-1, the word appended is too formal. A better choice is <u>attached</u>.

Cover letter 4

This letter includes a **paragraph on research highlights in five steps: topic, research gap/research niche*, findings, importance of the study** and **target audience**.

*Note: research gap/research niche

It is important to demonstrate the need for the research conducted. To do this, **authors refer to similar studies in the literature, focus on areas that have received little or no attention, and explain how their study fills the research gap and adds to what is currently known.** This is known as the **research gap** or **research niche**. Editors and reviewers pay considerable attention to justification of the relevance of research under review, and, for that reason, having **a clear and persuasive research gap/research niche is essential**.

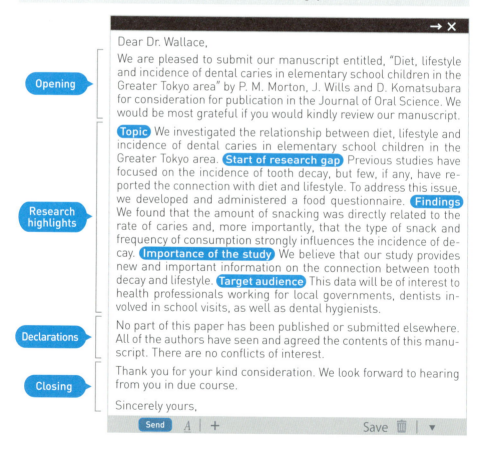

Opening
Dear Dr. Wallace,
We are pleased to submit our manuscript entitled, "Diet, lifestyle and incidence of dental caries in elementary school children in the Greater Tokyo area" by P. M. Morton, J. Wills and D. Komatsubara for consideration for publication in the Journal of Oral Science. We would be most grateful if you would kindly review our manuscript.

Research highlights
Topic We investigated the relationship between diet, lifestyle and incidence of dental caries in elementary school children in the Greater Tokyo area. **Start of research gap** Previous studies have focused on the incidence of tooth decay, but few, if any, have reported the connection with diet and lifestyle. To address this issue, we developed and administered a food questionnaire. **Findings** We found that the amount of snacking was directly related to the rate of caries and, more importantly, that the type of snack and frequency of consumption strongly influences the incidence of decay. **Importance of the study** We believe that our study provides new and important information on the connection between tooth decay and lifestyle. **Target audience** This data will be of interest to health professionals working for local governments, dentists involved in school visits, as well as dental hygienists.

Declarations
No part of this paper has been published or submitted elsewhere. All of the authors have seen and agreed the contents of this manuscript. There are no conflicts of interest.

Closing
Thank you for your kind consideration. We look forward to hearing from you in due course.
Sincerely yours,

Key sentences

Here is the same letter with the key sentences numbered. Each numbered sentence appears in the Quick Guide on page 24 with an explanation and further examples.

1. **We investigated** the relationship between diet, lifestyle and incidence of dental caries in elementary school children in the Greater Tokyo area.

2. **Previous studies have focused on** the incidence of tooth decay, **but few, if any, have reported** the connection with diet and lifestyle.

3. **To address this issue, we developed and administered** a food questionnaire.

4. **We found that** the amount of snacking was directly related to the rate of caries **and, more importantly**, that the type of snack and frequency of consumption strongly influences the incidence of decay.

5. **We believe that our study provides new and important information on** the connection between tooth decay and lifestyle.

6. **This data will be of interest to** health professionals **working for local governments, dentists involved in** school visits, as well as **dental hygienists**.

Quick Guide 4 »»»

In this quick guide, the key sentences from cover letter 4 are explained and further examples given.

1. State the topic　研究トピックの紹介

- <u>We investigated</u> the relationship between diet, lifestyle and incidence of dental caries in elementary school children in the Greater Tokyo area.

Explanation

The authors use the word **investigated** to introduce the main topic of the research. Notice that the active sentence using **we** is used.

Examples

- <u>We focused on</u> the relationship between diet, lifestyle and incidence of dental caries in elementary school children in the Greater Tokyo area.

In addition to **focused on**, other possible verbs are **investigated, looked at** and **studied**.

✎ Key Point

- Research highlights の書き出しは、'We investigated' や 'We focused on' を用いて研究テーマを簡単に説明する。

2. Describe the research gap/research niche
　　研究ギャップ・研究ニッチの説明

- <u>Previous studies have focused on</u> the incidence of tooth decay, <u>but few, if any, have reported</u> the connection with diet and lifestyle.

Explanation

There are two main steps. Firstly, the authors **refer to previous studies** using the following expression.

- <u>Previous studies have focused on</u> (+ topic).

The verbs **investigated** and **looked at** are commonly used.

Secondly, they state **areas of research that have received little or no attention** using the following expression.

- **but few, if any, have described/explored/investigated/reported** (subject/topic).

Other possible verbs are **concentrated on**, **looked at** and **reported on**.

Examples

Step 1 Refer to previous studies

- **There have been several studies on** the incidence of tooth decay.
- **A number of studies on** the incidence of tooth decay **have been published**.
- **Previous studies have focused on** the incidence of tooth decay.

Step 2 State the research gap

- **However, there is little in the literature on** (topic).
- **However, there have been few studies on** (topic).
- **However, to the best of our knowledge, there are no reports on** (topic).
- **However, research on X has been limited to** (topic).

Key Point

- 研究ギャップ／研究ニッチ（research gap/research niche）とは，まだ十分に研究されていないテーマのことをいう．
- 「○○についてはよく研究されている．しかし△△についてはまだよく分かっていない」の形で紹介するとよい．

3. State action taken　研究手法

- **To address this issue, we developed and administered** a food questionnaire.

Explanation

The authors refer to the issues raised in step 2 using the following phrase, **to address this issue**. Next, they mention the action taken using the words, **developed** and **administered**.

Examples

- **For that reason**, we developed and administered a food questionnaire.
- **Accordingly**, we developed and administered a food questionnaire.

🖉 Key Point

- 「△△についてはまだよく分かっていない．そこで…」という流れで，研究ギャップ・研究ニッチに続けて自分の研究を紹介するとよい．
- その際，'to address this issue' や 'for that reason' などの表現が便利である．

[4. Findings　研究結果]

- **We found that** the amount of snacking was directly related to the rate of caries **and, more importantly**, that the type of snack and frequency of consumption strongly influences the incidence of decay.

Explanation

The authors introduce the findings using the verb **found**. They stress the main point with the expression **and more importantly**.

Examples

- **Our results show that** snacking was directly related to the rate of caries **and, more importantly**, that the type of snack influences the incidence of decay.
- **The findings of this study suggest that** snacking was directly related to caries **and, more importantly**, that the type of snack influences the incidence of decay.
- **The results of this study indicate that** snacking was directly related to caries.

🖉 Key Point

- 研究結果は 'We found that (＋結果)' の形で説明する．
- 複数の結果を紹介するとき，より重要な結果を強調したいときには 'more importantly' を用いるとよい．

5. Importance of the study　研究の重要性

- <u>We believe that our study provides new and important information on</u> the connection between tooth decay and lifestyle.

Explanation

It is important to clearly state the new information presented in the paper and its significance for the field.

Examples

- <u>We consider that the findings reported here add important information to what is known about</u> lifestyle and early dental caries.
- <u>We believe that the findings bring new information to the field concerning</u> lifestyle and early dental caries.
- <u>In the opinion of the authors, the results presented here offer new insights on</u> lifestyle and early dental caries.
- <u>The authors believe that the results shed new light on the relationship between</u> lifestyle and early dental caries.

✏️ Key Point

- 'We believe' や 'We consider' を用いて論文の重要性をアピールするとよい。

6. Fit to the journal and relevance to readership
　　雑誌への適合性と想定読者層

- <u>This data will be of interest to</u> health professionals <u>working for local governments</u>, <u>dentists involved in</u> school visits, as well as <u>dental hygienists</u>.

Explanation

The authors use the expression **will be of interest to** in order to explain which groups of people will be interested in the paper.

Examples

- **This data will be useful for people working in the field of** community dentistry.
- **This data will be useful for people working on** ways of improving oral hygiene in very young children.
- **The findings presented here will be of direct practical interest to** a broad range of practicing dentists and researchers **in the field of** pedodontics.
- **The findings are relevant to** practicing dentists and researchers **in the field of** pedodontics.

Key Point

● 想定される読者層について説明するときは,'(研究結果／データ) will be of interest to (読者層)' の形を用いるとよい.

Notes on responding to reviewers' comments

3

Thanking reviewers
査読者への感謝の仕方

At the start of your replies to reviewers' comments, it is common to briefly express your thanks to the reviewer. I have noticed that some authors use very formal and sometimes dated English to do this.

Here are some examples.
×: *We deeply appreciate your fruitful comments and insightful suggestions.*
The above sentence is grammatically correct, but too formal and somewhat dated. A shorter and more neutral example is as follows:
○: *Thank you for your useful comments and suggestions.*

Another issue is that authors express their thanks too frequently. Here are some examples.

×: *Thank you for your comment. We have reduced the amount of data in Table 3.*

In this case, the change to the manuscript is small, and there is no need to thank the reviewer. A short response is all that is required. Here are two examples.

○: *We have reduced the amount of data in Table 3.*
○: *We have revised Table 3.*

Although it is not necessary to thank a reviewer for every comment, in some cases, where reviewers have made a comment or suggestion that has significantly improved the paper, authors may want to express their thanks. Here is an example.

○: *Thank you for drawing our attention to the errors in the statistical analysis.*

In this case, the authors are particularly grateful as the reviewer has noticed errors that might have been overlooked.

Here is another example.

○: *The reviewer suggested that we add a paragraph on the background to the study. We have done this and feel it improves the balance of the paper considerably. Thank you for the comment.*

Cover letter 5

In this section, I show how to answer questions listed in the instructions to authors. Here are some typical questions.

1. What questions does this work address?
2. How does this research add to existing knowledge?
3. For what reasons is this work important and timely?

Dear Dr. Walton,

We would be grateful if you would consider our manuscript entitled, "The role of exercise as an alternative treatment for depression and anxiety" by J. Ogata, L. C. Stuart and T. J. Williams for publication in the Journal of Mind and Health.

Below please find answers to the questions in the journal's instructions to authors.

Q1: What questions does this work address?

There have been a number of reports on the positive effects of exercise on depression and anxiety. However, it is not known which types of exercise are most effective. Additionally, there is little or no information on how exercise can be integrated with other treatments. We report the following: the effectiveness of different types of exercise, the degree to which symptoms are relieved, how long benefits continue, how exercise programs can be set up and maintained in institutions or the community, and also how they can be integrated with other approaches.

Q2: How does this research add to existing knowledge?

This research provides tentative answers to the question of which type of exercise is most effective in aiding recovery from depression and anxiety. It also provides data on the degree of improvement in patients who followed particular exercise programs, making comparisons about the effectiveness of different types of programs possible.

Q3: For what reasons is this work important and timely?

Since the positive effects of some medications for depression and anxiety are limited and cost is an issue, the results reported here may offer a solution to such problems, and for that reason, are important. The information may also encourage further research on alternative methods of treatment for depression and anxiety that are more cost effective, provide better results and offer other advantages.

We believe this work is timely because until recently there has been little research on alternative treatments for depression and, at the same time, there has been a growing interest in the positive effects of exercise on a number of mental illnesses.

The data presented has not been published, and is not currently being submitted for publication elsewhere. The work described here is original and all the authors have approved both the manuscript and this submission. We declare there are no conflicts of interest.

Thank you for considering our paper for review. We look forward to hearing from you in due course.

Sincerely yours,

Key Point

- 雑誌の投稿規定の中には，「研究ハイライト」に含めるべき事項について質問形式で問われていることがある．
- 投稿規定内の質問事項について，詳しくは Part 4（p.79 – 91）を参照．

Key sentences

Here is the same letter with the key sentences numbered. Each numbered sentence appears in the Quick Guide on page 34 with an explanation and further examples.

1. **Below please find answers to** the questions in the journal's instructions to authors.

Q1: What questions does this work address?

2. **There have been a number of reports on** the positive effects of exercise on depression and anxiety.

3. **However, it is not known** which types of exercise are the most effective.

4. **Additionally, there is little or no information on** how exercise can be integrated with other treatments.

5. **We report the following:** **the effectiveness of** different types of exercise, **the degree to which** symptoms are relieved, **how long** benefits continue, **how** exercise programs **can be set up and maintained** in institutions or the community, and also **how they can be integrated** with other approaches.

Q2: How does this research add to existing knowledge?

6. **This research provides tentative answers to the question of** which type of exercise is most effective in aiding recovery from depression and anxiety. **It also provides data on** the degree of improvement in patients who followed particular exercise programs, **making comparisons about** the effectiveness of different types of programs **possible**.

Q3: For what reasons is this work important and timely?

7. **Since** the positive effects of some medications for depression and anxiety **are limited and cost is an issue, the results reported here may offer a solution to** such problems, **and for that reason, are important. The information may also encourage further research on** alternative methods of treatment for depression and anxiety that are more cost effective, provide better results and offer other advantages.

8. **We believe this work is timely because** until recently **there has been little research on** alternative treatments for depression and, at the same time, **there has been a growing interest in** the positive effects of exercise on a number of mental illnesses.

Quick Guide 5 >>>

In this quick guide, the key sentences from cover letter 5 are explained and further examples given.

1. The authors introduce their answers to the questions in the Instructions to Authors　投稿規定内の質問事項に回答する

- <u>Below please find answers to</u> the questions in the journal's instructions to authors.

Explanation

It is important to clearly introduce your answers to the questions listed in the Instructions to Authors.

Examples

- <u>Please find below answers to the questions posed in the journal's Instructions to Authors</u>. 1.　2.　3.（show a numbered list of responses）
- <u>The following are our answers to the questions in the journal's Instructions to Authors</u>. 1.　2.　3.（show a numbered list of responses）
- <u>Our responses to questions in the guidelines for authors are as follows</u>: 1.　2.　3.（show a numbered list of responses）

✏️ Key Point

● はじめに，これから投稿規定内の質問事項に回答することをはっきり示すとよい．

3. Research gap: Known information　研究ギャップ：はじめに既知の事実について述べる

- <u>There have been a number of reports on</u> the positive effects of exercise on depression and anxiety.

Explanation

An important part of establishing a research gap is to refer to what is known about a topic.

Examples

- **It has been reported that** exercise relieves some of the symptoms of depression and anxiety.
- **It has been widely reported that** exercise relieves some of the symptoms of depression and anxiety.
- **It is known that** exercise relieves some of the symptoms of depression and anxiety.
- **We know that** exercise relieves some of the symptoms of depression and anxiety.
- **A number of studies have reported/shown that** depression and anxiety are relieved by exercise.
- **A number of authors have reported/stated that** depression and anxiety are relieved by exercise.

[**3. Research gap: Unknown information (1)**
研究ギャップ：未解明の研究課題を紹介する(1)]

- **However, it is not known** which types of exercise are most effective.

Explanation

Here the authors focus on areas of the field that have received little or no attention.

Examples

- **However, we do not know** which types of exercise are the most effective.
- **However, it is unknown** which types of exercise are the most effective.
- **However, little is known about** which types of exercise are the most effective.
- **Previous studies have focused on** exercise programs to relieve stress, **but little is known about** which types of exercise are the most effective.

[**4. Research gap: Unknown information (2)**
研究ギャップ：未解明の研究課題を紹介する(2)]

- **Additionally, there is little or no information on** how exercise can be integrated with other treatments.

Explanation

The authors continue to create the research gap by stating areas of the research field that have received little or no attention.

Examples

- **Also, little is known about** the benefits and how long they continue.
- **In addition, there have been no studies on** the benefits and how long they continue.
- **There has been little research on** the benefits and how long they continue.
- **To date, no reports have been published on/concerning** the benefits and how long they continue.
- **To the best of our knowledge, there have been no reports on** the benefits and how long they continue.

In the following example, the above three steps for explaining a research gap/niche are combined.

① **Known information**
② **Unknown information (1)**
③ **Unknown information (2)**

- ①**It has been widely reported that** exercise relieves some of the symptoms of depression and anxiety. ②**However, we do not know** which types of exercise are most effective. ③**Additionally, there is little or no information on** how exercise can be integrated with other treatments.

[
5. The authors state the main focus of the study
研究の概要を説明する
]

- **We report the following**: **the effectiveness of** different types of exercise, **the degree to which** symptoms are relieved, **how long** benefits continue, **how** exercise programs **can be set up and maintained** in institutions or the community, and also **how they can be integrated** with other approaches.

Explanation

The authors briefly list the main points investigated.

Examples

- **We investigated the following:** (list of the points investigated)
- **We looked at the following:** (list of the points investigated)
- **We focused on the following:** (list of the points investigated)

🖉 Key Point

● 研究テーマに関する質問に対しては，①既知の事実→②研究ギャップ→③研究の概要，という順番で回答するとよい．

---

6. State how the information reported adds to existing knowledge　この研究がどのような新知見をもたらすかを説明する

- **This research provides tentative answers to** the question of which type of exercise is most effective in aiding recovery from depression and anxiety. **It also provides data on** the degree of improvement in patients who followed particular exercise programs, **making comparisons about** the effectiveness of different types of programs **possible**.

Explanation

It is important to stress what is new and how your research adds to what is already known about the topic.

Examples

- **The findings reported here give possible answers to** the question of which type of exercise is the most effective.
- **These findings add to what we know about** alternative ways of aiding recovery from depression.

🖉 Key Point

● この研究によって既存の知識に何が追加されるのかを，'provide' や 'add' などの動詞を使って説明する．

7. Explain the importance of the data　研究結果の重要性を説明する

- <u>Since</u> the positive effects of some medications for depression and anxiety <u>are limited and cost is an issue, the results reported here may offer a solution to</u> such problems, <u>and for that reason, are important</u>. <u>The information may also encourage further research on</u> alternative methods of treatment for depression and anxiety that are more cost effective, provide better results and offer other advantages.

Explanation

First, the authors refer to an issue in the field.

- <u>Since</u> the positive effects of some medications for depression and anxiety <u>are limited, and cost is an issue,</u> (this sentence is continued below)

Next, they mention how their results offer a solution.

- <u>the results reported here may offer a solution to</u> such problems, <u>and for that reason, are important</u>.

Following that, they mention how the research affects the field.

- <u>The information contained here may also encourage further research on</u> alternative methods of treatment for depression and anxiety that are more cost effective, provide better results and display other advantages.

Examples

1. Refer to an issue in the field

- <u>Considering</u> the various limitations associated with current medications and treatments for depression and anxiety, (this sentence is continued below)

2. Explain how the reported findings offer solutions to outstanding issues

- <u>the findings reported here provide useful</u> solutions to the problem.

3. Explain how the research affects the field

- <u>The findings may also promote interest in</u> a previously under-researched alternative treatment.

8. Give reasons why the work is important and timely
この研究がタイムリーである理由を説明する

- <u>We believe this work is timely because until recently there has been little research on</u> alternative treatments for depression and, at the same time,<u> there has been a growing interest in</u> the positive effects of exercise on a number of mental illnesses.

Explanation
The authors introduce their answer to **question 3**:
For what reasons is this work important and timely?

Examples

- <u>We consider this research to be timely because</u> until recently <u>there has been little research on</u> alternative treatments for depression.
- <u>This research is timely because</u> until recently <u>there have been few studies on</u> alternative treatments for depression.

🖉 Key Point
- 研究の重要性・タイムリー性に関する質問に対しては，当該研究分野における問題点や課題を指摘したうえで，この研究がその解決につながることを説明するとよい．

Notes on responding to reviewers' comments

4

Words with the prefix re
接頭辞're'で始まる言葉

Have you noticed how frequently the prefix <u>re</u> is used in responses to reviewers' comments? Here are some examples.

1. When you make changes to the text, these words are frequently used: **rephrase**, **rewrite**, **reword**.
   - The sentence at the bottom of page 17 **has been rephrased**.
   - We **have rewritten** the Discussion section.
   - The title **has been reworded** to reflect the importance of the participants' feedback.

2. When talking about the structure of a paper, the following words are frequently used: **reorganize** and **restructure**. Here are some examples.
   - The Discussion **has been reorganized** to stress the importance of the new measurement system.
   - The Conclusion **has been restructured** so as to emphasize the main points.

3. Other useful words are as follows: **reanalyze**, **recalculate**, **redraw**, **replot**, **rework**. Here are some examples.
   - The data from experiments 1 and 2 **has been reanalyzed**.
   - The statistical analysis on page 17 **has been recalculated**. No changes to the text have been made.
   - Figure 3 has been **redrawn** to make it easier to see the melting peak and transition.
   - The graph showing the melting peak **has been replotted**.
   - The Introduction **has been reworked** taking into account the comments made by both reviewers.

Part 2
Cover letters for submission of revised manuscripts

A cover letter is useful when submitting a revised manuscript as editors can see how authors have responded to the main issues raised by the reviewers. Authors should state that they are submitting a revised version of a previously submitted manuscript, giving the date of the original submission, the reference number and a brief explanation of responses to major issues raised. A detailed list of all the changes to the manuscript should be attached separately. Below you will find four example cover letters.

1. Basic cover letter with no explanation of responses to reviewers' comments

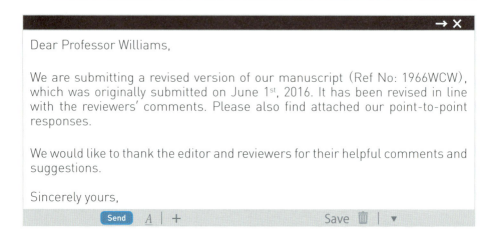

Dear Professor Williams,

We are submitting a revised version of our manuscript (Ref No: 1966WCW), which was originally submitted on June 1st, 2016. It has been revised in line with the reviewers' comments. Please also find attached our point-to-point responses.

We would like to thank the editor and reviewers for their helpful comments and suggestions.

Sincerely yours,

Key sentences

1. We are submitting a revised version of our manuscript (Ref No: 1966WCW), which was originally submitted on June 1st, 2016.

2. It has been revised in line with the reviewers' comments.

3. Please also find attached our point-to-point responses.

4. We would like to thank the editor and reviewers for their helpful comments and suggestions.

Key Point

- 査読者による指摘を受けて論文を修正した後，修正原稿（改訂稿）を再投稿する際も，必要事項を記入したカバーレターを用いる．
- この例のように，必要最小限の事項だけを記入したシンプルなカバーレターを用いてもよい．
- あるいは，次ページ以降の例のように，主な修正点についてカバーレター中で説明してもよい．

2. Cover letter that includes a brief description of the main changes to the manuscript

Dear Professor Simms,

We are submitting a revised version of our manuscript (Ref No: 1966WCW), which was originally submitted on June 1st, 2016. The main changes are as follows:
1) We have revised the Introduction and included a more detailed literature review.
2) We have extended the Methods section and included several new Tables showing how experiments were performed.
3) Finally, we have reduced the conclusion by a page and listed the main findings so as to improve readability.

Please find attached our point-to-point responses to the reviewers' comments, and a revised copy of the manuscript with changes shown in red. We trust that the revised manuscript will meet with the approval of the editor and reviewers. We very much appreciate the helpful comments and suggestions made by the reviewers.

Sincerely yours,

Key sentences

1. <u>We are submitting a revised version of our manuscript</u> (Ref No: 1966WCW), **which was originally submitted on** June 1st, 2016.

2. <u>The main changes are as follows</u>: (show a numbered list of the major changes)

3. <u>Please find attached our point-to-point responses to the reviewers' comments, and a revised copy of the manuscript with changes shown in red.</u>

4. <u>We trust that the revised manuscript will meet with the approval of the editor and reviewers.</u>

5. <u>We very much appreciate the helpful comments and suggestions made by the reviewers.</u>

Quick Guide 6 »»

This quick guide focuses on key sentences from cover letters 2.1 and 2.2 for submission of revised manuscripts.

[
1. State you are submitting a revised manuscript
修正原稿の再投稿であることを述べる
]

- **We are submitting a revised version of our manuscript** (Ref No: 1966WCW), **which was originally submitted on** June 1st, 2016.

Explanation

The authors state they are submitting a revised version of their manuscript, and give the reference number and date of submission.

Examples

- **We wish to submit a revised version of our manuscript** (Ref No: 1966WCW), **which was originally submitted on** June 1st, 2016.
- **We wish to submit our revised manuscript entitled**, "The effects of exercise programs on institutionalized adults with mild dementia", **which was originally submitted on** (date) **and has the following reference number** (ref. no.).
- **I am attaching a revised version of our paper entitled**, "The effect of lifestyle changes on residents of carehomes by P. M. Morton, N. Suzuki and K. Watanabe", **which was originally submitted on** September 22, 2015. **The reference number is** KUMB1916.
- **We are submitting our revised manuscript entitled**, "The effect of lifestyle changes on residents of carehomes by P. M. Morton, N. Suzuki and K. Watanabe", **which was originally submitted on** September 22, 2015. **The reference number is** KUMB1916.
- **Please find attached our revised manuscript entitled**, "The effect of lifestyle changes on residents of carehomes by P. M. Morton, N. Suzuki and K. Watanabe", **which was originally submitted on** September 22, 2015. **The reference number is** KUMB1916.

📝 Key Point

- 修正原稿の再投稿時のカバーレターも，書き出しは初回投稿時と同様に 'Please find attached' などの表現を用いる．
- 修正原稿（a revised version）であることを明記したうえで，論文受付番号と初投稿年月日（＋タイトル，著者名）も示す．

2. Refer to revisions made in the manuscript
修正を行ったことを述べる

- **It has been revised in line with the reviewers' comments**.

Explanation

It is common to briefly refer to how you have dealt with reviewers' comments.

Examples

- **All of the reviewers' comments/suggestions have been reflected/incorporated in the revised manuscript**.
- **As far as possible, we have revised the manuscript in line with the reviewers' comments**.
- **Where possible, we have revised the manuscript in line with the reviewers' comments**.

📝 Key Point

- はじめに，査読者の指摘どおりに修正を行ったことを説明するとよい．

3. Introduce a brief summary of the main changes
主な修正点を簡潔に説明する

- **The main changes are as follows: (1) We have revised** the Introduction and included a more detailed literature review. (2) **We have extended** the Methods section and included several new Tables showing how experiments were performed. (3) **Finally, we have reduced** the Conclusion by a page **and listed the main findings** so as to improve readability.

Explanation
Here the authors refer to extensive changes and give concrete examples.

Examples

- <u>**Based on the comments of the three reviewers, we have made substantial changes to our manuscript as follows:**</u> (show a numbered list of the main changes)
- <u>**The following is a brief summary of the main changes to the manuscript.**</u> (show a numbered list of the main changes)
- <u>**The main changes are as follows:**</u> (show a numbered list of the main changes)

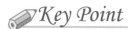Key Point

● 主な修正点については，その概要を箇条書きで示す．

---

4. Refer to the list of detailed responses
修正内容の詳細なリストを添付したことを述べる

- <u>**Please find attached**</u> our point-to-point responses to the reviewers' comments.

Explanation
Most authors state that a detailed list of responses and corrections is attached.

Examples

- <u>**We have attached our point-to-point responses separately**</u>.
- <u>**Detailed responses to the reviewers' comments are attached**</u>.
- <u>**We have attached a list of all the changes made in/to the manuscript**</u>.

Key Point

● 査読者の全指摘事項に対する詳細な返答については，別ファイルにまとめるとよい．
● カバーレターでは，返答リストを添付したことを説明すればよい．

5. State that the revised manuscript is attached
修正原稿が添付されていることを述べる

- Please find attached our point-to-point responses to the reviewers' comments, **and a revised copy of the manuscript with changes shown in red**.

Explanation
The authors state that a revised manuscript is attached.

Examples
- **The revised manuscript with changes shown in red is attached**.
- **We have attached the revised manuscript. Changes are in red**.

Key Point
- 修正原稿を添付したことを説明する．
- 修正原稿では，修正箇所は赤で示すようにすると，どこを修正したのかが分かりやすい．

6. Thank the editor and reviewers
編集者と査読者への感謝を述べる

- **We very much appreciate the helpful comments and suggestions made by the reviewers**.

Explanation
It is usual to finish the letter by thanking the editor and reviewers.

Examples
- **Thank you for your useful comments on our paper**.
- **We wish to thank the editor and reviewers for their critical comments**.
- **We would like to thank the reviewers for their helpful advice and suggestions**.
- **We would like to thank the reviewers for carefully reading our manuscript and providing us with useful comments and suggestions**.
- **We would like to thank the reviewers for their helpful advice and suggestions**.
- **We wish to thank the reviewers for their useful comments, which have done a lot to improve the quality of our manuscript**.

- Finally, we would like to thank the editor and reviewers for their comments, which have greatly helped to improve the quality of the manuscript.
- We appreciate the time the reviewers have spent on our paper.
- We feel the paper has been much improved as a result of the reviewers' comments and suggestions.
- We wish to thank the editor and reviewers for their valuable comments, which we believe have resulted in a much improved manuscript.
- We would like to express our gratitude to the editor and reviewers for their helpful comments and suggestions, which have improved our manuscript.

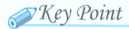

Key Point

- 最後に，編集者と査読者への感謝を述べるようにする．

5 Notes on responding to reviewers' comments

How do you handle a reviewer's comment that is unclear?

査読コメントが不明瞭なときはどうすればよいのか？

Editors and reviewers who are non-native speakers of English probably outnumber those who are native speakers. Inevitably, there will be times when the quality of English in comments to authors will be variable. In some cases, quality will be poor and communication difficult. The following question arises: What do you do when you cannot understand a reviewer's comment? Here are some useful expressions to be used when you cannot follow exactly what point the reviewer is making.

In these three examples, the authors <u>summarize the reviewer's comment as they understand it</u>. They then respond.

- <u>*If we understand correctly, the reviewer would like to know about*</u> *the sampling methods and reasons for excluding several sites. (followed by a response)*
- <u>*We assume that the reviewer is asking about*</u> *the sampling methods and reasons for excluding several sites. (followed by a response)*
- <u>*We take it that the reviewer is asking about*</u> *the sampling methods and reasons for excluding several sites. (followed by a response)*

How to confirm a question

- <u>*We would like to confirm the meaning of the reviewer's comment. Is the reviewer asking about*</u> *the sampling methods and reasons for excluding several sites? If so, our answer is as follows: (show response)*
- <u>*We find this comment difficult to understand. Is the reviewer asking about*</u> *the sampling methods and reasons for excluding several sites? If so, our answer is as follows: (show response)*

3 Cover letter including detailed explanations of the main changes to the manuscript (1)

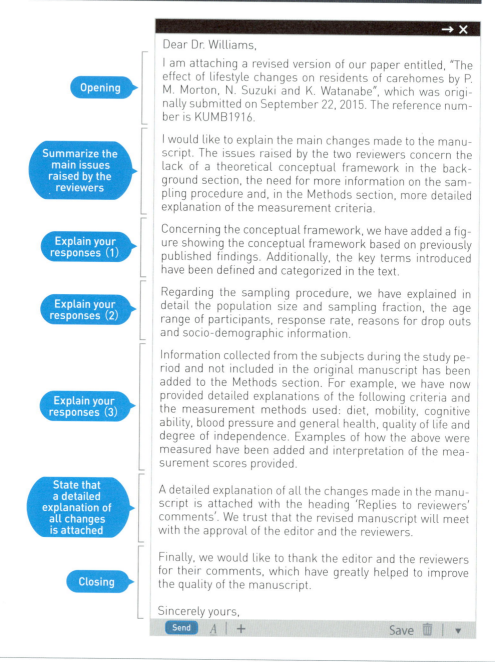

Opening

Dear Dr. Williams,

I am attaching a revised version of our paper entitled, "The effect of lifestyle changes on residents of carehomes by P. M. Morton, N. Suzuki and K. Watanabe", which was originally submitted on September 22, 2015. The reference number is KUMB1916.

Summarize the main issues raised by the reviewers

I would like to explain the main changes made to the manuscript. The issues raised by the two reviewers concern the lack of a theoretical conceptual framework in the background section, the need for more information on the sampling procedure and, in the Methods section, more detailed explanation of the measurement criteria.

Explain your responses (1)

Concerning the conceptual framework, we have added a figure showing the conceptual framework based on previously published findings. Additionally, the key terms introduced have been defined and categorized in the text.

Explain your responses (2)

Regarding the sampling procedure, we have explained in detail the population size and sampling fraction, the age range of participants, response rate, reasons for drop outs and socio-demographic information.

Explain your responses (3)

Information collected from the subjects during the study period and not included in the original manuscript has been added to the Methods section. For example, we have now provided detailed explanations of the following criteria and the measurement methods used: diet, mobility, cognitive ability, blood pressure and general health, quality of life and degree of independence. Examples of how the above were measured have been added and interpretation of the measurement scores provided.

State that a detailed explanation of all changes is attached

A detailed explanation of all the changes made in the manuscript is attached with the heading 'Replies to reviewers' comments'. We trust that the revised manuscript will meet with the approval of the editor and the reviewers.

Closing

Finally, we would like to thank the editor and the reviewers for their comments, which have greatly helped to improve the quality of the manuscript.

Sincerely yours,

Key sentences

1. I would like to explain the main changes made to the manuscript.

2. **The issues raised by the two reviewers concern** the lack of a theoretical conceptual framework in the background section, **the need for more information on the sampling procedure and, in the Methods section, more detailed explanation of** the measurement criteria.

3. Concerning the conceptual framework, we have added a figure showing the conceptual framework based on previously published findings.

4. Additionally, the key terms introduced have been defined and categorized in the text.

5. Regarding the sampling procedure, we have explained in detail the population size and sampling fraction, the age range of participants, response rate, reasons for drop outs and socio-demographic information.

6. Information collected from the subjects during the study period and not included in the original manuscript has been added to the Methods section.

7. For example, we have now provided detailed explanations of the following criteria and the measurement methods used: diet, mobility, cognitive ability, blood pressure, general health, quality of life and degree of independence.

8. Examples of how the above were measured have been added and interpretation of the measurement scores provided.

9. A detailed explanation of all the changes made in the manuscript is attached with the heading 'Replies to reviewers' comments'.

10. We trust that the revised manuscript will meet with the approval of the editor and the reviewers.

Notes on responding to reviewers' comments

6

How long does it take to revise and resubmit a paper?
修正原稿の再投稿までにどのくらい時間をかけるか？

Everything will depend on the type and number of comments you receive from the reviewers. Comments that require minor changes to the text such as adding or deleting information can be dealt with easily and quickly. Some comments will require you to write longer responses where you justify an approach, finding or conclusion. Time is, of course, a key factor and most authors will be eager to resubmit their paper and start work on something else. In fact, many authors try to avoid writing extensive responses involving justifications and so on. In some cases, the simplest solution is to delete the part of the text that is an issue. Of course, this might not always be possible, but it is certainly one solution that may save you a lot of time.

Quick Guide 7 »»

In this quick guide, the key sentences from cover letter 2.3 are explained and further examples given.

1. Introduce the main changes　主な修正点の紹介

- <u>I would like to explain the main changes made to the manuscript</u>.

<u>Explanation</u>

The above sentence signals the start of your explanation of how you have handled the main issues raised by the reviewers.

<u>Examples</u>

- <u>I have addressed the reviewers' concerns as outlined below</u>.（show a numbered list of major revisions）
- <u>Below you will find our responses to the main concerns raised by the reviewers</u>.（show a numbered list of major revisions）
- <u>Our responses to the main points made by the reviewers are explained below</u>.（show a numbered list of major revisions）
- <u>We have dealt with the major points raised by the reviewers as follows</u>:（show a numbered list of major revisions）

✎ Key Point

● はじめに，主な修正点について説明することを述べる．

2. Restate the criticism made by the reviewers
　　査読者からの指摘事項の要約

- <u>The issues raised by the two reviewers concern</u> the lack of a theoretical conceptual framework in the background section, <u>the need for</u> more information on the sampling procedure <u>and, in the Methods section, more detailed explanation of</u> the measurement criteria.

<u>Explanation</u>

Firstly, you should briefly summarize the reviewer's main criticisms.

Examples

- **Reviewer 2 was concerned about** the lack of a control group.
- **The reviewers were concerned about** the length of the manuscript.
- **The reviewers raised concerns about** the length of the manuscript.
- **Reviewer 1 expressed concerns about** the lack of a control group.
- **Both reviewers were critical of** the sampling techniques.
- **Reviewer 1 commented that** a theoretical conceptual framework **is necessary and should be included in** the Introduction.

NOTE:

In examples 1 and 2 above, **was concerned** and **were concerned** can be in the **present tense** as follows: **is concerned, are concerned**. Also in example 5, **were critical** can be **are critical**. In these examples, it is possible to use either the past or present tense.

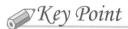Key Point

- 修正点を説明するにあたって、まず査読者の指摘を要約して示すとよい。
- 査読者の指摘に言及するときは 'concern' 'comment' などの動詞を用いる。

3. Explain the changes made to the manuscript (1)　修正点の説明(1)

- **Concerning the conceptual framework, we have added** a figure showing the conceptual framework based on previously published findings.

Explanation

The issue raised by the reviewer is introduced with the expression, **concerning the conceptual framework**. The word **concerning** is used to introduce a topic. The action taken by the authors is briefly introduced using the expression **we have added**. It would also be possible to use the expression **we added**. Other expressions similar to **concerning** are as follows: **as for, regarding, with regard to**.

Examples

- **As for the conceptual framework, we have added** a figure showing the conceptual framework based on previously published findings.
- **Regarding the conceptual framework, we have added** a figure showing the conceptual framework based on previously published findings.
- **With regards to the conceptual framework, we have added** a figure showing the conceptual framework based on previously published findings.

Key Point

- 修正点を説明する文章は，'Concerning（＋査読者の指摘事項）'などの表現で書き始めるとよい．
- 修正点の説明は，現在完了形（we have added）／過去形（we added）のどちらを用いてもよい．

4. Explain the changes made to the manuscript (2)　修正点の説明 (2)

- **Additionally, the key terms introduced have been defined and categorized in the text**.

Explanation

The author's response to a connected issue raised by the reviewer is introduced with the word **additionally**. Action taken by the authors is introduced with the phrase **X has/have been defined and categorized**.

Examples

- **We have also added** a Table to the Methods section.

5. Explain the changes made to the manuscript (3)　修正点の説明 (3)

- **Regarding the sampling procedure, we have explained in detail** the population size and sampling fraction, the age range of participants, response rate, reasons for drop outs and socio-demographic information.

Explanation

This response is introduced with the phrase **regarding** (+ topic). New information added to the text is introduced with the phrase, **we have explained in detail** (+ information).

Examples

- **To address the problem of reliability, we have provided details of** the population size and sampling fraction.
- **To address the question of the sampling procedure, we have shown in detail** the population size and sampling fraction.
- **As for the issue of reliability,** detailed information on the population size and sampling fraction **has been added to the manuscript**.

6. Explain the changes made to the manuscript (4)　修正点の説明 (4)

- **Information collected from the subjects during the study period and not included in the original manuscript has been added to the Methods section**.

Explanation

The authors explain how more data has been added.

Examples

- **We have added more information on** the subjects in the Methods section.
- **We have included more information on** the subjects in the Methods section.
- **More information on the subjects has been included in** the Methods section.

7. Explain the changes made to the manuscript (5)　修正点の説明 (5)

- **For example, we have now provided detailed explanations of the following criteria and the measurement methods used**: diet, mobility, cognitive ability, blood pressure, general health, quality of life and degree of independence.

Explanation

The verb **provide** is used to explain what has been added.

Examples

- **More detailed information has been added** concerning measurement methods.
- **More detailed information has been provided** concerning measurement methods.
- **Detailed information has been provided** in terms of measurement methods.

8. Explain the changes made to the manuscript (6)　修正点の説明(6)

- **Examples of how the above were measured have been added and interpretation of the measurement scores provided**.

Explanation

The verbs **added** and **provided** are used to introduce changes to the manuscript.

Examples

- **We have added examples of how the above were measured, and also provided interpretation of the measurement scores**.
- **Information on** measurement methods and **interpretation of scores has been added**.

9. Refer to the list of detailed changes
　　詳細な修正内容のリストを添付したことの説明

- **A detailed explanation of all the changes made in the manuscript is attached with the heading 'Replies to reviewers' comments'**.

Explanation

The authors state that a detailed list of all the changes made in the manuscript is attached. The word **attached** is used.

Examples

- <u>We are attaching a detailed explanation of all the changes made in the manuscript with the heading, 'Replies to reviewers' comments'</u>.
- <u>A detailed list of changes to the manuscript is attached</u>.
- <u>A detailed explanation of all the changes made is attached</u>.
- <u>Point-by-point replies to reviewers' comments are attached</u>.
- <u>Detailed replies to the reviewers' comments are attached</u>.

10. Closing　結びの挨拶

- <u>We trust that the revised manuscript will meet with the approval of the editor and the reviewers</u>.

Explanation

Here are some examples of how to finish your explanation of the main changes made to the text.

Examples

- <u>We hope that the above changes to the manuscript will meet with the approval of the editor and the reviewers</u>.
- <u>We trust that the revisions made to the manuscript will be acceptable to the editors and reviewers</u>.

Key Point

● 修正点についての説明は，上記のような表現で締めるとよい．

Notes on responding to reviewers' comments

7

Comments concerning the quality of English
英語の質について指摘されたらどうすればよいか？

In some cases, editors and reviewers criticize the quality of English in a paper and make general comments that seem to be unjustified. For example, the following criticisms are common.

- *The English is poor and should be revised.*
- *The quality of the English in this paper does not meet the standards of the journal.*
- *There are a number of language issues that need attention.*

If you are confident in the quality of English in your manuscript, and it has been professionally edited, the following response may be useful. It should be used only in cases where you feel the reviewers' comments are unjustified.

Concerning the critical comments on the quality of English in our manuscript, we would respectfully point out that it has been checked by a professional editor and two native-speakers of English, both of whom are familiar with the field. In the opinion of the authors, the English in this paper is acceptable. If the reviewers would kindly provide us with examples of where our English is incorrect, we would gladly make the necessary changes. As it stands, we feel that further revision is unnecessary.

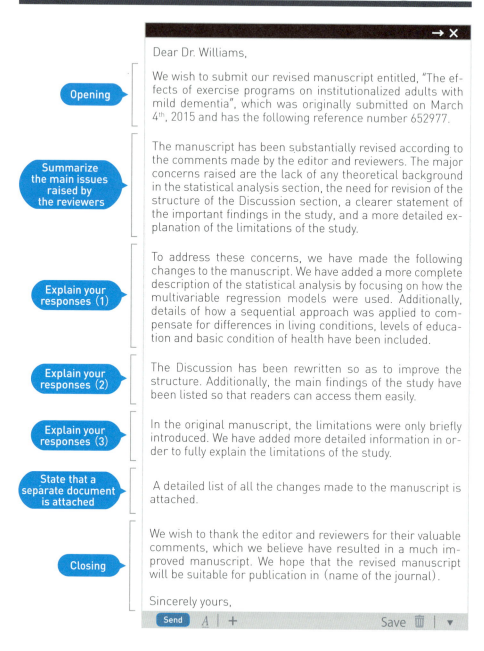

Key sentences

1. The manuscript has been substantially revised according to the comments made by the editor and reviewers.

2. The major concerns raised are the lack of any theoretical background in the statistical analysis section, **the need for** revision of the structure of the Discussion section, **a clearer statement of** the important findings in the study **and a more detailed explanation of** the limitations of the study.

3. To address these concerns, we have made the following changes to the manuscript.

4. We have added a more complete description of the statistical analysis by focusing on how the multivariable regression models were used. Additionally, **details of** how a sequential approach was applied to compensate for differences in living conditions, levels of education and basic condition of health **have been included**.

5. The Discussion has been rewritten so as to improve the structure. **Additionally, the main findings of the study have been listed so that** readers can access them easily.

6. In the original manuscript, the limitations were only briefly introduced. **We have added more detailed information** in order to fully explain the limitations of the study.

7. We hope that the revised manuscript will be suitable for publication in (name of the journal).

Quick Guide 8 »»»

In this quick guide, the key sentences from cover letter example 2.4 are explained and further examples given.

[1. Statement concerning revisions made 修正を行ったことを述べる]

- The manuscript has been substantially revised according to the comments made by the editor and reviewers.

Explanation

In the cover letter, you should explain your responses to the major issues raised by the reviewers.

Here I list 5 verbs that can be used when referring to revisions made. Verbs 1 and 2 refer to minor changes and verbs 5 and 6 to major changes.

- This paper has been **1. modified** in line with the reviewers' comments.
  - **2. altered**
  - **3. changed**
  - **4. revised**
  - **5. substantially revised**
  - **6. completely rewritten**

Examples

- The manuscript has been completely rewritten based on the reviewers' comments.
- The manuscript has been revised on the basis of the comments made by the editor and reviewers.

✎ Key Point

● 修正を行ったことを述べる際、修正が比較的軽微な場合には 'modified' や 'altered' を、全面的な大修正の場合には 'substantially revised' や 'completely rewritten' を用いるとよい。

2. Restatement of the reviewers' major concerns
査読者の主な指摘を要約する

- **The major concerns raised are the lack of** any theoretical background in the statistical analysis section, **the need for** revision of the structure of the Discussion section, **a clearer statement of** the important findings in the study **and a more detailed explanation of** the limitations of the study.

Explanation

It is usual to summarize the reviewers' main criticisms using the following expression,

- **The major concerns raised by the editor and the reviewers are as follows:** (followed by a list of numbered points)

The word **concerns** could be changed to **issues** or **points**. The word **raised** is frequently used with **concerns** and **issues**. For example:

- **The major concerns raised** are as follows: (followed by a list of numbered points)
- **The major issues raised** are as follows: (followed by a list of numbered points)

Examples

- **The reviewers pointed out the following issues in the manuscript.**
- **The main issues raised by the reviewers are as follows**: (followed by a list of numbered points)
- **The reviewers raised the following issues.** (followed by a list of numbered points).
- **Major criticisms raised by the reviewers are as follows**: (followed by a list of numbered points)

🖋 Key Point

● 査読者の主な指摘事項を挙げる際は，'The major concerns/issues/points raised are as follows:' の後に続けるとよい．

3. State your responses to the main issues raised by the reviewers
査読者の主な指摘に対する対応を述べる

- <u>To address these concerns, we have made the following changes to the manuscript</u>.

Explanation

The above sentence is used to signal the start of the authors' responses to the issues raised.

Examples

- <u>We have revised our manuscript according to the points raised by the reviewers</u>.
- <u>We have changed our manuscript in line with the comments made by the reviewers</u>. **The main revisions are as follows**. (followed by a list of numbered points)
- <u>To address the issues raised, the following changes have been made to the manuscript</u>. (followed by a list of numbered points)

🖉 Key Point

● 査読者の指摘への対応を説明する際は，その合図として上記のような文章を用いるとよい．

4. Statement of main changes in detail　主な修正点を詳しく説明する

- <u>We have added</u> a more complete description of the statistical analysis by focusing on how the multivariable regression models were used. **Additionally**, **details of** how a sequential approach was applied to compensate for differences in living conditions, levels of education and basic condition of health **have been included**.

Explanation

The authors start to explain in detail the main changes made to the manuscript. Both active and passive structures are used with the verbs **add** and **include**. **We have added** (active), **X have been included** (passive).

Examples

- **We have revised the description of the statistical analysis by focusing on how** the multivariable regression models were used.
- **We have provided details of** the multivariable regression models that were used.

🖉 Key Point

● 修正内容を説明するときは,受動態と能動態のどちらを用いてもよい.

5. Statement of action taken（1）　修正点を説明する（1）

- **The Discussion has been rewritten** so as to improve the structure. **Additionally, the main findings of the study have been listed** so that readers can access them easily.

Explanation

The authors state the changes made to the manuscript using the verbs, **rewritten** and **listed**.

Examples

- **We have revised the Introduction and added several new references**.
- **The Discussion has been reduced by** two paragraphs.

6. Statement of action taken（2）　修正点を説明する（2）

- **In the original manuscript, the limitations were only briefly introduced. We have added more detailed information in order to fully explain the limitations of the study**.

Explanation

The authors restate the problem, **In the original manuscript, the limitations were only briefly introduced.** Then, they explain the changes made. **We have added more detailed information in order to fully explain the limitations of the study.** The expression **in the original manuscript** refers to the manuscript as it was first submitted.

Examples

- **Concerning the limitations**, more detailed information has been added.
- **Regarding the limitations**, more detailed information has been added.
- **As for the limitations**, more detailed information has been added.
- **With regard to the limitations**, more detailed information has been added.

7. Closing the cover letter　結びの挨拶

- **We hope that the revised manuscript will be suitable for publication in** (name of the journal).

Explanation

The authors finish the cover letter with the sentence **We hope that the revised manuscript will be suitable for publication in** (name of the journal).

Examples

- **We trust that our manuscript is suitable for publication in** (name of the journal).
- **We very much hope that the manuscript will be acceptable for publication in** (name of the journal).

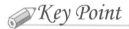Key Point

- カバーレター全体の結びとして，論文採択への思いを記すのもよい．

Part 3
Research Highlights

On page 10, I explained the origin of research highlights in academic papers and their use in cover letters for initial and revised submissions. In cover letters 2 ~ 5, pages 10 to 39, I provided examples of research highlights ranging from three to five steps containing the following topics, **research niche**, **methods**, **findings**, **importance of the paper** and **target audience**. Here I introduce an example of **detailed research highlights**, which can be used in both **cover letters** and **pre-submission inquiries**. On the following page, you will find it broken down into sections with subheadings that explain the functions. There is also an explanation of the sentences, expressions and vocabulary used.

1 Example of detailed research highlights
研究ハイライトの例

We looked at the effectiveness of preventive programs in reducing the risk of cognitive decline in groups of people over the age of 60 living in carehomes. In the UK, there are almost 1 million people suffering from cognitive impairment, and treatment costs are in the region of 30 billion pounds yearly. We focused on the following research questions: (1) What factors are important in the creation of preventive programs? (2) How much improvement can be expected? (3) Which of the elements in a preventive program is the most significant?

There have been a number of reports on how cognitive decline in the elderly may be linked to lifestyle factors, but no studies have focused on how preventive programs can reduce mental decline. This study is the first to address how a preventive program focusing on regular exercise, smoking cessation, dietary advice and maintaining a healthy heart can limit cognitive decline.

Results of tests on program participants showed that post-program scores were 20 percent higher than pre-program, with improvements in spatial awareness, thought processes and cognitive abilities. Considering the increased number of people with dementia, the huge costs involved, and limited success in research on new drugs, preventive programs are promising in terms of outcome and cost. We believe this manuscript is appropriate for publication in the Journal of the Aged in Society because it addresses issues that currently affect healthcare services worldwide, and reports on the essential elements of a successful preventive program. It will be of particular interest to those involved in the design, implementation and administration of similar preventive programs.

2 Detailed research highlights: analysis of the main functions

研究ハイライトの構成

Here each section of the above research highlights has a heading for the purposes of explanation. These are shown in blue.

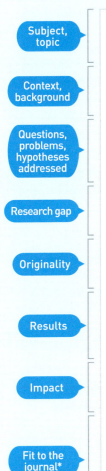

Subject, topic: We looked at the effectiveness of preventive programs in reducing the risk of cognitive decline in groups of people over the age of 60 living in carehomes.

Context, background: In the UK, there are almost 1 million people suffering from cognitive impairment, and treatment costs are in the region of 30 billion pounds yearly.

Questions, problems, hypotheses addressed: We focused on the following research questions: (1) What factors are important in the creation of preventive programs? (2) How much improvement can be expected? (3) Which of the elements in a preventive program is the most significant?

Research gap: There have been a number of reports on how cognitive decline in the elderly may be linked to lifestyle factors, but no studies have focused on how preventive programs can reduce mental decline.

Originality: This study is the first to address how a preventive program focusing on regular exercise, smoking cessation, dietary advice and maintaining a healthy heart can limit cognitive decline.

Results: Results of tests on program participants showed that post-program scores were 20 percent higher than pre-program, with improvements in spatial awareness, thought processes and cognitive abilities.

Impact: Considering the increased number of people with dementia, the huge costs involved, and limited success in research on new drugs, preventive programs are promising in terms of outcome and cost.

Fit to the journal*: We believe this manuscript is appropriate for publication in the Journal of the Aged in Society because it addresses issues that currently affect healthcare services worldwide, and reports on the essential elements of a successful preventive program. It will be of particular interest to those involved in the design, implementation and administration of similar preventive programs.

*Note:

'Fit to the journal' refers to the match between the aims and scope of the journal and the contents of the paper submitted.

3.1,3.2 Example of detailed research highlights

3. Analysis of the sentences, expressions and vocabulary used in the above example

研究ハイライトの各要素の解説

1. Subject/topic 研究テーマ・トピック

- <u>We looked at</u> the effectiveness of preventive programs in reducing the risk of cognitive decline in groups of people over the age of 60 living in carehomes.

Explanation

The authors introduce the subject of their research with the expression, **We looked at** (topic). It is also possible to use these expressions: **We focused on** (topic), **We studied** (topic). More formal expressions are as follows: **We investigated** (topic), **We examined** (topic). The verbs **examined**, **investigated** and **studied** are commonly used in the passive. For example, (Topic) **was examined/investigated/studied**. The verbs **look at** and **focus on** are almost always used in the active tense. For example, **We looked at** (topic). **We focused on** (topic).

🖉 Key Point

- 研究テーマは 'investigate' 'focus on' 'look at' などを用いて紹介する.
- 能動態でも受動態でもどちらでもよいが，受動態でよく使われる動詞と能動態でよく使われる動詞は異なるので注意する.

2. Context/background 背景

- <u>In the UK, there are almost 1 million people suffering from cognitive impairment, and treatment costs are in the region of 30 billion pounds yearly</u>.

Explanation

The authors provide background by stating basic factual information concerning the topic. Notice that verbs are in the present tense and the language is simple.

🖉 Key Point

- 研究の背景となる事実を，簡潔に，現在形で説明する.

3. Questions/problems/hypotheses addressed
   検証した問題・疑問・仮説

- **We focused on the following questions**: (1) What factors are important in the creation of preventive programs? (2) How much improvement can be expected? (3) Which of the elements in a preventive program is the most significant?

Explanation

The authors introduce their research questions with the sentence, **We focused on the following questions**. The questions are numbered, which makes them more direct and easier to follow. The questions themselves are simple.

The following three examples can also be used.

- **In this study, the questions/problems we wanted to investigate were as follows**: (1) What factors are important in the creation of preventive programs? (2) How much improvement can be expected? (3) Which of the elements in a preventive program is the most significant?
- **We hypothesized that** preventive programs focusing on diet and exercise **would reduce** cognitive decline in old people, and **posed the following questions**: (1) What factors are important in the creation of preventive programs? (2) How much improvement can be expected? (3) Which of the elements in a preventive program is the most significant?
- **Cognitive decline is considered to be a serious issue in institutionalized adults. We wanted to see if exercise could help relieve symptoms, and set out to answer the following questions**: (1) What factors are important in the creation of preventive programs? (2) How much improvement can be expected? (3) Which of the elements in a preventive program is the most significant?

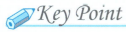Key Point

- この研究がどのような疑問・仮説を検証したのか，箇条書きで列挙する．

4. Research gap　研究ギャップ（未研究分野・範囲）の指摘

- <u>There have been a number of reports on</u> how cognitive decline in the elderly may be linked to lifestyle factors, <u>**but no studies have focused on**</u> how preventive programs can reduce mental decline.

Explanation

To establish the **research gap**, the authors firstly refer to **topics that have been studied** (Step 1).

Examples Step 1 (These sentences are continued below in Step 2)

- <u>There have been a number of reports on/concerning</u> （+ topic）.
- <u>Several studies have focused on</u> （+ topic）. <u>See, for example</u>, Smith (2016).
- <u>A number of studies have looked at</u> （+ topic）. <u>See, for example</u>, Smith (2016).

Next, the authors introduce **areas of research that have received little or no attention** (Step 2).

Examples Step 2

- <u>but no studies/few studies/a limited number of studies have focused on</u> （+ topic）.
- <u>but there have been few reports on</u> （+ topic）.
- <u>but little is known about</u> （+ topic）.

Here is an example that combines steps 1 and 2 above in one sentence.

- <u>Several studies have focused on</u> general preventive programs, <u>but little is known about</u> the positive effects of a combined exercise program.

✏️ Key Point

- 研究ギャップについて、「すでに分かっていること→まだ分かっていないこと」の順に説明する。
- 研究ギャップ（研究ニッチ）については、p. 24, p. 34, p. 84 も参照。

5. Originality　独創性

- <u>**This study is the first to address how**</u> a preventive program focusing on regular exercise, smoking cessation, dietary advice and maintaining a healthy heart can limit cognitive decline.

Explanation

The authors stress the originality of the submission with the expression, This study is the first to **address** how（topic）.
Other possible verbs are **consider, describe, evaluate, examine, focus on, investigate, look at, report**.

Examples

- <u>**To the best of our knowledge, this is the first study to focus on**</u> the effect of exercise on mental decline.
- <u>**To our knowledge, this is the first study on**</u> the effect of exercise on mental decline.
- <u>**We show for the first time how a preventive program focusing on**</u> regular exercise, smoking cessation, dietary advice and maintaining a healthy heart <u>**can prevent cognitive decline.**</u>
- <u>**This study is the first to demonstrate that**</u> regular exercise, smoking cessation, dietary advice and maintaining a healthy heart <u>**may be effective as a therapy for cognitive decline.**</u>

The verb **demonstrate** can be changed to **show, report** or **prove**.

🖉 Key Point

● 研究の独創性については，「○○について調べたのはこの研究が初めてである」のような形でアピールするとよい．

6. Results　結果

- <u>Results of tests on</u> program participants <u>showed that</u> post-program scores were 20 percent higher than pre-program, with improvements in spatial awareness, thought processes and cognitive abilities.

Explanation

Here the main findings are described using the verb **showed**. Other verbs are as follows: **confirm, demonstrate, indicate, suggest**. The verb **suggest** is weaker than the others.

Examples

- Results from tests of mobility <u>**confirm**</u> the benefits of an exercise program.
- A slowing in the rate of cognitive decline <u>**demonstrated**</u> the benefits of the program.
- Results <u>**indicate/suggest**</u> that exercise slowed cognitive decline.

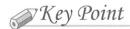*Key Point*

○ 研究結果を 'show' 'confirm' 'demonstrate' などを用いて紹介する。

7. Impact　研究分野へのインパクト

- <u>Considering</u> the increased number of people with dementia, the huge costs involved, and <u>limited success</u> in research on new drugs, <u>preventive programs are promising in terms of</u> outcome and cost.

Explanation

The authors explain how the findings of their study have an impact on the field. They start by explaining the current situation.

- <u>**Considering the increased number of people with dementia**</u>, the huge costs involved, <u>**and limited success in research on**</u> new drugs, (this sentence is continued below)

The authors then explain why preventive programs are promising.

- **preventive programs are promising in terms of** outcome and cost.

Examples

- **Taking into account** the relative lack of success in treating some cases of dementia, **the current approach offers** a useful additional therapy.
- **In terms of** the relative lack of success in treating some cases of dementia, **programs focusing on exercise and lifestyle changes may present** useful additional therapies.
- **Considering** the relative lack of success in treating some cases of dementia, **the results presented here are useful as they demonstrate/show/suggest the potential of lifestyle changes in slowing dementia**.

Key Point

● 研究分野に与えるインパクトを説明するには，①研究分野における問題点・課題を述べる→②この研究がその解決に寄与することを示す，の2段構成を用いるとよい．

8. Fit to the journal　雑誌への適合性

- **We believe this manuscript is appropriate for publication in** (journal name) **because it addresses** issues that currently affect healthcare services worldwide, and **reports on** the essential elements of a successful preventive program. **It will be of particular interest to** those involved in the design, implementation and administration of similar preventive programs.

Explanation

The authors introduce the fit to the journal. In the first sentence, they explain **how the manuscript matches the aims and scope of the journal**. In the second sentence, they mention **the target audience**.

Examples

1. How the manuscript matches the aims and scope of the journal

- <u>We think this paper is suitable for publication in</u> (journal name) <u>because it focuses on issues</u> that currently affect healthcare services worldwide.
- <u>We consider that this research fits the aims of the journal and also meets the needs of the readership</u> since <u>it looks at</u> issues affecting healthcare services worldwide, <u>and is relevant to those working in the field of</u> community dentistry.
- <u>This paper is a good match to the journal as it focuses on</u> issues that currently affect healthcare services worldwide.

2. Fit to the target audience

- <u>This paper will appeal to researchers/people working in the field of community dentistry.</u>
  <u>This paper will be of interest to researchers/people working on community health projects.</u>
- <u>This research will interest those involved in</u> the planning and implementation of community health programs.

🖉 Key Point

● 論文が投稿先の雑誌にマッチしていることを，①雑誌の目的・対象範囲との合致，②論文の想定読者層，の2点からアピールする．

Part 4
How to handle questions concerning research highlights

Most journals include questions concerning research highlights in Instructions to Authors. These depend on the journal but generally cover a narrow range of topics, five of which are listed below. The purpose of this section is to provide model answers to such questions.

1. Subject, topic, context, background : One or two sentences stating the subject/topic. In some cases, you should also include information on the context and background.
2. Research gap, originality : A statement explaining the research gap that stresses the originality of the study.
3. Importance of the results : A statement outlining the main results and their importance.
4. Impact on the field : A statement explaining how the results affect what is already known about the field.
5. Fit to the journal : A statement explaining how the manuscript fits the scope of the journal and the readership.

Model answers for questions in categories 1 ~ 5 are shown below. Authors will probably need to answer several of these questions depending on the journal.

1 Subject, topic, context, background
研究テーマ・背景

In this section, I look at the following five sentences.

What subject/topic did you investigate?
What is the context/background of this work?
What is the rationale?
What issues led to this work?
What problems/questions/hypotheses does this research address?

1.1 What subject/topic did you investigate? 研究テーマは何か?

This question can be answered in the following way.

- **We looked at/focused on** the link between cognitive decline in aged people and risk factors such as diet, blood pressure and levels of physical activity.

Here the informal verb **looked at** can be used. It is also possible to use **focused on, investigated, researched, studied**.

In more formal English, the word **we** can be omitted and the sentence changed from active to passive. Here is an example.

- The link between cognitive decline in aged people, and risk factors such as diet, blood pressure and levels of physical activity **was investigated**.

1.2 What is the context/background of this work? この研究の背景は何か?

Question 1.2 focuses on the context/background of the study. Unlike question 1.1, it cannot be answered in one sentence, since more information is needed.

- In the aged population, **later-life cognitive impairment and dementia is increasing. Human, social and economic costs are becoming serious issues. One promising approach is** prevention, **particularly interventions such as diet, exercise and other lifestyle changes**.

The above paragraph can be divided into three main functions as follows:

1. Summary of known facts about the topic

- In the aged population, **later-life cognitive impairment and dementia is increasing**.

2. Analysis of wider issues

- **Human, social and economic costs are becoming serious issues**.

3. Introduction of possible solutions

- **One promising approach is** prevention, **particularly** interventions **such as** diet, exercise and other lifestyle changes.

[1.3 What is the rationale?　この研究を行った動機は？]

Similar questions are as follows:
What is the reason for this study?
What is the need for this study?

- **Since** later-life cognitive impairment and dementia, as well as associated costs, are increasing, **the need for solutions is pressing**. **The main purpose of this work is to** identify factors that may prevent cognitive decline.

There are two main functions here.

1. Statement of known facts

- **Since** later-life cognitive impairment and dementia, as well as associated costs, are increasing, **the need for solutions is pressing**.

2. Statement of the main purpose of the study

- **The main purpose of this work is to** identify factors that may prevent cognitive decline.

1.4 What issues led to this work?
どのような問題を解決するためにこの研究を行ったのか？

This question is similar to question 1.3 and focuses on the reasons for the research.

- <u>It is estimated that</u> one third of people may suffer from some form of dementia in their lives, and this presents a considerable challenge for healthcare services. <u>Research on</u> interventions such as diet and exercise <u>is promising</u>, and <u>further research work is required</u>.

There are three main functions here.

1. Statement of known facts

- <u>It is estimated that</u> one third of people may suffer from some form of dementia in their lives,

2. How the above fact presents a problem

- <u>and this presents</u> a considerable challenge for healthcare services.

3. How the current study presents a possible solution

- <u>Research on</u> interventions such as diet and exercise <u>is promising</u>, and <u>further research work is required</u>.

1.5 What problems/questions/hypotheses does this research address?
この研究はどのような問題・疑問・仮説を検証したのか？

Here, authors are required to list the problems, questions or hypotheses that their research addresses.

- <u>We addressed the question of whether</u> preventive programs <u>could be effective in reducing cognitive decline. We posed the following questions</u>:
  <u>1. How far can lifestyle changes prevent dementia</u>?
  <u>2. How important is diet</u>?
  <u>3. To what extent does physical exercise help</u>?

To answer the questions in 1.5, three steps are required.

1. State the research problem/question/hypothesis

- **We addressed the question of** whether preventive programs could be effective in reducing cognitive decline.
- **We looked at the question of** whether preventive programs could be effective in reducing cognitive decline.

2. Signal the start of the research questions

- **We posed the following questions**: (list of research questions)
- **Our main research questions are as follows**: (list of research questions)
- **We focused on the following research questions**: (list of research questions)

3. List the research questions

- **1. How far can lifestyle changes prevent dementia?**
  2. How important is diet?
  3. To what extent does physical exercise help?

Here are examples using the words **hypothesize** and **hypothesis**.

- **We hypothesized that prevention programs focusing on** lifestyle changes such as diet and exercise **would be effective in reducing cognitive decline**, and **set up** a series of experiments **to investigate the effectiveness of** such a program.
- **Our main hypothesis was that** prevention programs **focusing on** lifestyle changes such as diet and exercise **would be effective in reducing** cognitive decline, and **set up** a series of experiments **to investigate the effectiveness** of such a program.

🖉 Key Point

- 研究テーマに関する質問に対しては，'focus on' 'look at' などを用いて回答する．
- 研究の背景や理由に関する質問には，その研究分野における課題・問題点を紹介したうえで，自分の研究がその解決につながることを示せばよい．

2 Research gap/originality

研究ギャップ・独創性

For more information on research gaps, see page 24.
In this section, I focus on the following five questions.

Questions 2.1 ~ 2.3 focus on **research topics that have received little attention**. This is known as **the research gap**.
2.1 What is not previously published?
2.2 What area has not previously been studied?
2.3 What is the gap being filled?

Questions 2.4 ~ 2.5 focus on **originality**.
2.4 What is new? What is different? What is the novelty of this work?
2.5 How is this work original?

To answer the questions in section 2, a 3-step structure is necessary. Steps 1 and 2 concern the research gap and step 3 focuses on originality.

Research gap
Step 1 Refer to previously published work on the same topic
Step 2 State areas that are under-researched
Steps 1 and 2 relate to the research gap. Step 1 mentions work already done on the same topic, and is important because it is related to the under-researched areas introduced in step 2.

Originality
Step 3 State how your work is original
Step 3 is a statement of the originality of the work.

Here are some examples of each of the three steps.

> **Step 1: Refer to previously published work on the same topic**
> はじめに, 同テーマの先行研究について述べる

- <u>A number of studies have focused on</u> cognitive decline in later-life individuals.
- <u>A lot/much has been written about</u> cognitive decline in later-life individuals.
- Cognitive decline in later-life individuals <u>is well reported</u>.
- Cognitive decline in later-life individuals <u>has received considerable/a lot of attention</u>.
- <u>There have been a number of studies on</u> cognitive decline in later-life individuals.

Step 2: State areas that have been under-researched
次に, まだ未解明の研究課題を紹介する

- **However, preventive programs remain under-researched**.
- **However, there have been no reports/studies on** preventive programs.
- **But no published studies have investigated** the benefits of preventive programs.
- **But there have been no published results on** the benefits of preventive programs.
- **But there have been few studies on** the benefits of preventive programs.
- **But the benefits of** preventive programs **have not been reported**.

Note: Steps 1 and 2 can be written as either one or two sentences.

Step 3: State how your work is original
最後に, この研究の独創性・新規性について述べる

- **This study/work/research is innovative/original because it focuses on/demonstrates** ways of reducing dementia cases.
- **Here we report a new method for** reducing the number of dementia cases.
- **The main novelty of this research is that it assesses** several preventive programs.

Here is an example using the three steps explained above.

Step 1 Cognitive decline in later-life individuals **has received a lot of attention** in recent years. **Step 2** **However, few studies have focused on** the benefits of preventive programs involving light exercise and other lifestyle changes. **Step 3** **In this paper, we report** the establishment of a program involving comprehensive exercise therapy, and **give details of** improvements in cases of mild dementia.

🖊 Key Point

● 研究ギャップ, 研究の独創性に関する質問に対しては, ①先行研究への言及→②まだ分かっていないことの紹介→③自身の研究の独創性・新規性の紹介, の3段構成で回答するとよい.

3 Importance of the work
研究の重要性

In this section, I focus on the following questions.

What are the major results/overall findings/most important conclusions?
Why is the novel content mentioned above important?
Why is this research important and timely?

3.1 What are the major results/overall findings/most important conclusions? 主な結果・発見・結論は何か？

Question 3.1 is the easiest to answer because it simply requires a statement of the main results/findings/conclusions. Here are some examples.

- <u>The main results are as follows:</u>
  (1) Dietary interventions slow the symptoms of dementia
  (2) Single nutrients have limited effects
  (3) Combinations of nutrients bring memory improvements in patients in the early stages of the disease
- <u>The most notable results are as follows:</u> (show a numbered list of results)
- <u>The main conclusions are as follows:</u> (show a numbered list of main conclusions)
- <u>The following is a summary of the main conclusions of the study.</u> (show a summary of the main conclusions)

3.2 Why is the novel content mentioned above important? その結果は，どのように重要なのか？

It is necessary to explain the importance of the novel content. Here are some example sentences.

- <u>These results are important in terms of</u> the potential of alternative treatments for dementia.
- <u>These results are important because they prove</u> the potential of alternative treatments for dementia.
- <u>These results present solid evidence that</u> alternative methods can play a crucial role in treatments.

- **These results are important because they provide a new way** to treat dementia.
- **The findings reported here are important because they show that** mental decline can be slowed by dietary and exercise intervention.
- **The data provided here is important because it proves that** mental decline can be relieved by dietary and exercise intervention.
- **These results are important because they advance our knowledge of/improve our understanding of** preventive programs.

3.3 Why is this research important and timely?
この研究が重要でタイムリーである理由は何か？

Importance of the research

- **These results are important because previously it was unclear how** mental decline can be relieved by lifestyle changes.
- **These results are important because they show how** dietary intervention can improve care of the elderly in the community.
- **It is important to clarify** the potential of this intervention and, **for that reason, the results presented here are important**.
- **The results presented here are important for the following reasons:** (show a list of numbered points)

Timeliness of the research

- **This work is timely because it shows that** the symptoms of dementia can be relieved by lifestyle changes.
- **These results are timely, particularly in terms of** the recent government report on care for the elderly in the community.
- **These results are timely because** of the current work on dementia prevention.
- **There are several reasons why this study is timely:** (show a list of numbered points)

Key Point

● 研究の重要性に関する質問に対しては，主な研究結果を紹介したうえで，それが重要である理由・タイムリーである理由を説明するとよい．

4 Impact on the field
研究分野へのインパクト

In this section, I focus on the following questions.

What is the potential impact on the field?
How does this paper advance our current understanding of this field?
How do these results and conclusions fit in with what is known about the field?

4.1 What is the potential impact on the field?
この論文は，この研究分野にどのようなインパクトを与えるか？

- Although interventions in terms of diet, exercise and other lifestyle factors have been tried in patients showing signs of early dementia, **there have been few reports in the literature on** the effect of different types of exercise. **This is the first time that data from a number of alternative approaches have been compared**. **We consider that the results reported here will** promote research on various alternative interventions.

4.2 How does this paper advance our current understanding of this field? この論文は，この分野の現在の知見をどのように広げるか？

- **These results add to our current understanding of** how light exercise can be used as an additional treatment for early cognitive decline.
- **These results impact on our current understanding of** how light exercise can be used as an additional treatment for early cognitive decline.
- **These results have an impact on our current understanding of** how light exercise can be used as an additional treatment for early cognitive decline.
- **Previously, we knew that** exercise was a potentially useful method in the fight against mental decline, **but there were no reports on** the extent of benefits or the type of exercise. **We now know that** a combination of treatments is beneficial.

4.3 How do these results and conclusions fit in with what is known about the field?　この研究の結果は，この分野における既存の知識とどのように関連するか？

- <u>**The key findings of this study are listed below. We believe these will have a significant impact on the field since**</u> they have previously received little or no attention.（show a numbered list of key findings）
- <u>**One of the most important conclusions from this research is the fact that it shows**</u> how exercise programs can reduce the rate of mental decline in people with mild symptoms.
- <u>**We consider that our results add to existing knowledge of**</u> possible alternative treatments.

🖉 Key Point

- 自分の研究が研究分野に与えるインパクトについて，既存の知識との関連をもとに説明するとよい．

5 Fit to the journal
雑誌への適合性

In this section, I focus on the following five questions.

How the research matches the journal
5.1. How does this research fit in with the scope and aims of this journal?
5.2. Why does this work belong in this journal?
5.3. How will this paper benefit the journal?

How the research fits the readership
5.4. How does this work fit the readership?
5.5. Why will this work appeal to readers of this journal?

Questions 5.1 ~ 5.3 relate to the way in which the manuscript matches the journal. Questions 5.4 ~ 5.5 refer to the readership.

5.1 How does this research fit in with the scope and aims of this journal?
この研究は,この雑誌の対象範囲・目的にどのように合致するか?

- <u>Since the majority of readers of this journal are involved in community health initiatives, the results reported here will be of interest as they provide details of</u> the effectiveness of dietary interventions that could be used in community health situations.
- The findings presented here indicate the effectiveness of dietary intervention, <u>**and are therefore relevant to the scope of this journal**</u>.

5.2 Why does this work belong in this journal?
この研究は,この雑誌にどのように適しているか?

- <u>We believe this manuscript is appropriate for publication in</u> (journal name) <u>because the findings increase our understanding of the effectiveness</u> of dietary interventions.

> **5.3 How will this paper benefit the journal?**
> この論文は,この雑誌にどのようなメリットをもたらすか？

- <u>This journal has published a number of papers on</u> lifestyle interventions, <u>a topic that is attracting considerable attention</u>. <u>Our paper reports the effect of diet and exercise interventions, and adds to what has already been published in the journal</u>.
- <u>We consider that our findings will/can contribute to research on</u> lifestyle interventions for people with mild cognitive decline, <u>and, for that reason, will benefit the journal</u>.

Here questions 5.4 and 5.5 **refer to the readership**.

> **5.4 How does this work fit the readership?**
> この研究は,この雑誌の読者層とどのようにマッチしているか？

- <u>We think the findings reported here contribute to our understanding of</u> alternative treatments for dementia, <u>indicate</u> the benefits derived from such programs, <u>and are therefore relevant to the readership.</u>

> **5.5 Why will this work appeal to readers of this journal?**
> この研究は,この雑誌の読者にとってどのように魅力的か？

- <u>The results reported here will be of interest to people involved in</u> community health initiatives, and <u>that includes the design, implementation, and evaluation of those programs</u>.

✏️ Key Point

● 自分の論文が投稿先の雑誌に適合していることをアピールするためには、雑誌の対象範囲や読者層と自分の研究との関連を示すとよい.

Notes on responding to reviewers' comments

8

Apologizing

査読者への感謝は必要か？

In responses to reviewers' comments, authors apologize too frequently, sometimes using very formal English. Below I show several examples of this problem, and provide suggestions for revision.

1. ×:*We regret to say that we have no data.*
 → ○:*We have no data on that topic.*
    ○:*We are unable to provide that data.*
    ○:*Unfortunately, we cannot provide that data.*
    ○:*It is not possible to provide that data, as it is classified.*

2. ×:*Sorry about the Conclusion. There are too many sentences.*
 → ○:*We agree that the Conclusion is too long, and have deleted several sentences.*
    ○:*We have revised the Conclusion and reduced it in length by 10 lines.*

3. ×:*I'm sorry about the mistake on page 7.*
 → ○:*The mistake on page 7 has been corrected.*
    ○:*We have corrected the mistake on page 7.*
    ○:*We have rectified the problem on page 7.*
    ○:*We have addressed the issue on page 7.*

Part 5
Responding to reviewers' comments

In this section, I focus on highly frequent responses to reviewers' comments, which I have divided into seven categories as follows:

1. Simple revisions
2. Comments concerning language
3. Requests for more information
4. Clarifying a point
5. Explaining why you cannot comply with a reviewer's request
6. Explaining why you do not want to make a suggested change
7. Responding to critical comments

1 Simple revisions
軽微な修正を求めるコメントへの対応

Here I give examples of how to handle simple changes to the manuscript.

Comment 1 軽微な修正を求めるコメント①

Page 7, line 25. The notation used in this equation is incorrect.

Response

- **Thank you for pointing out this error**. The notation **has been changed as follows**: (show revised version)

Explanation

The reviewer points out a small but significant error. From the response, **Thank you for pointing out this error**, it is clear that the authors are grateful the reviewer has noticed the error.

Examples

Examples 1 and 2 are formal and use academic vocabulary.

1. Thank you for **drawing this problem to our attention**. **The notation has been changed as follows**. (show revised version)

The academic verb **draw something to someone's attention** is used. The second sentence is passive, **has been changed**, which creates a detached, formal style.

2. Thank you for **bringing this point to our attention**. **The notation has been revised as follows**. (show revised version)

The academic verb **bring something to someone's attention** is used. In addition to the word **point,** it would be possible to use **mistake, error, problem** or **issue**. The words **problem** and **issue** are usually used for serious matters.

Examples 3 and 4 below are less formal.

3. **We have changed the notation**. **It now reads as follows:** (show revised version)
4. **We have changed the notation, which is now as follows:** (show revised version)

Responses 3 and 4 are short. The authors do not thank the reviewer. There is no use of formal, academic vocabulary. Both examples use the active tense, **we have changed**.

In examples 1 and 2, the authors thank the reviewers. They do this because the error might have been missed. However, it is **unnecessary to thank the reviewers for every comment**. For more information on **Thanking**, see **Notes on responding to reviewers' comments 3**, page 28.

Short response

In part 5 of this book, I provide examples of the shortest possible responses.

- **The notation has been changed**.
- **We changed the notation**.

Key Point

- 単純ミスなどの軽微な指摘に対しては，査読者への感謝の言葉はなくてもよい（査読者への感謝の仕方については p. 28 のコラムを参照）．
- 修正したことを述べる際は 'have changed' などの表現を用いる．

Comment 2　軽微な修正を求めるコメント②

There are a number of problems in the list of references. For example in reference 17, the year seems to be incorrect. The references should be checked.

Response

- The year **is incorrect**. **It should be** 2003. We have revised the manuscript accordingly.
- **This is a mistake**. The reference **should be** 2003. We have checked all of the references and made revisions where necessary.

Explanation

The author admits the mistake and corrects the error using the pattern **should be**.

- **It should be** (show revised version).
- **The reference should be** (show revised version).

5.1 Simple revisions

Examples

- Mistakes in the reference list **have been corrected**.
- We have checked the reference list and **made a number of corrections as follows**: (show revised version)
- **We have made the necessary changes to the list of references**.
- **We have changed the list of references accordingly**.

Short response

- **We have revised the references**.
- **The references have been revised**.

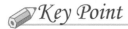Key Point

● 単純な誤りに言及するときは，'should be' という表現も便利である。

[Comment 3　軽微な修正を求めるコメント③]

Some of the calculations made in the data analysis section are incorrect. The figures should be checked.

Response

- **We apologize for** the errors made in the data analysis section. **These have been corrected in the revised manuscript**. **Corrections are shown in red**.

Explanation

The authors apologize for the errors and state that the necessary corrections have been made.

Examples

- **As pointed out, there were several errors in** the data analysis section. **These mistakes have been corrected/changed/rectified in the revised manuscript, and are shown in red**.
- **The errors in the data analysis section have been corrected**.

Short response

- **The data analysis has been checked. Revisions are in red**.

Comment 4　軽微な修正を求めるコメント④

What is the origin of the pollution? How did it get into the water?

Response

- In the original manuscript, **we incorrectly stated that** the water was polluted. **The word pollution has been deleted from the manuscript**.

Explanation

The phrase, **we incorrectly stated that**, is used to refer to the error. The action taken is introduced with the phrase, **X has been deleted**.

Examples

- **There was an error** in the original manuscript. **We incorrectly stated that** the water was polluted. **The manuscript has been revised accordingly**. (show revised version)
- **Our statement that** the water was polluted **was incorrect**. **This problem has been addressed**. (show revised version)
- **There was a mistake** in the original manuscript. **We incorrectly stated** that the water was polluted. **This issue has been dealt with**. (show revised version)

Short response

- **We have deleted** the word pollution.

🖉 Key Point

● 誤った記述について言及するときは 'We incorrectly stated that'，それを削除するときは 'has been deleted' を用いるとよい．

5.1 Simple revisions

> **Summary**
>
> **Simple revisions**
> 軽微な修正を求めるコメントへの対応
>
> Frequently used sentence patterns are as follows:
>
> - The notation **has been changed** as follows:(show revised version)
> - **We have changed** the notation. It now **reads as follows**:(show revised version)
> - X **is incorrect**. **It should be** (show revised version).
> - The errors in the data analysis section **have been corrected**. The revised version now **reads as follows**:(show revised version)
>
> Frequently used verbs are as follows:
> **altered, changed, corrected, deleted, rectified, revised, rewritten, should be.**
> The verb **read** is used to indicate the revised version. For example: **The revised version reads as follows**:(show revised version)
>
> - 軽微な修正について説明するときは'altered''changed''corrected'などの表現を用いる。
> - 修正後の文章を示すときは'The revised version reads as follows:'の後に続けるとよい。

Notes on responding to reviewers' comments

9

How short can responses to reviewers' comments be?
査読コメントへの返答は,どのくらい短くてもよいのか?

Let's take a look at four different responses to the following reviewer's comment.

Comment
Please delete the last sentence on page 7 of the manuscript.

Example responses
1. *We have deleted the sentence.*
2. *We deleted the sentence.*
3. *Deleted.*
4. *Done.*

As mentioned on page 117, <u>Notes on responding to reviewers' comments 10</u>, there is a slight difference in formality between the present perfect tense, <u>have deleted</u>, and the simple past tense, <u>deleted</u>, with the former being more formal and polite. Although in many cases in this book, I have stated that the shortest response is usually the best, I feel that examples 3 and 4 are too direct. They consist of single verbs, <u>deleted</u> and <u>done</u>. The word done is generally considered to be informal. For me, the shortness and informality of the sentences make them too direct, and I would hesitate to recommend these forms for use in responses to reviewers' comments. I would add, however, that I recently saw a number of responses to reviewers' comments that consisted of a single word only. The following words were used: <u>added</u>, <u>defined</u>, <u>deleted</u>, <u>fixed</u>, <u>omitted</u>, <u>rewritten</u>, <u>revised</u>. These one word responses were in Minor revisions. Sometimes, authors might have a large number of comments concerning minor revisions to deal with and, in that case, one word responses may be appropriate.

2 Comments concerning language
英語の質に関するコメントへの対応

This section focuses on how to respond to comments concerning language.

> **Comment 1**　英語の質に関するコメント：論文全体についての指摘

There are a large number of grammar and syntax errors.

Response

- The manuscript **has been edited by a native speaker of English. Corrections in the revised manuscript are shown in red.**

Explanation

In this case, the reviewer does not refer to specific errors, and the authors do not give examples of revisions made. They simply state that the manuscript has been professionally edited.

Examples

- **The manuscript has been edited by** a native speaker of English from a company providing professional English editing services.
- **This paper has been proofread by** a native speaker.
- **The manuscript has been edited by an experienced editor specializing in papers on** ophthalmology.
- **The manuscript has been checked by** two coworkers proficient in English and familiar with the field.
- **A native speaker of English has checked** the manuscript.

In example 5, the sentence is active and the verb **checked** is less formal than **edited, proofread** or **revised**.

🖉 Key Point

- 論文全体の英語の質に関して，具体的に欠くコメントを受け取った場合は，英文校正を受けたことを伝えればよい．
- その際は 'edited' 'proofread' などの表現を用いる．

Comment 2　英語の質に関するコメント：具体的な箇所についての指摘

Page 3, line 15. This sentence is unclear and should be revised.

Response

- **We have revised the sentence as follows**:（show revised sentence）

Explanation

This comment refers to a specific sentence, but not to a particular grammatical or lexical error. The authors state that the sentence has been revised.

Examples

- **We have rewritten/changed/reworded** this sentence. **It now reads as follows**:（show revised sentence）

🖉 Key Point

● 修正の必要がある場合には，'We have revised the sentence as follows:' などの表現に続けて，修正後の文章を示せばよい．

Summary — Comments concerning language　英語の質に関するコメントへの対応

Frequently used sentence patterns are as follows:

- **This manuscript has been revised by** a native speaker of English.
- **This manuscript has been edited by** a native speaker of English.
- **This paper has been proofread by** a native speaker.
- **A native speaker of English has revised this paper**.
- **The revised sentence/version is as follows**:（show revised version）
- **We have reworded the title, which is as follows**.（show revised title）
- **We have reworded the title. The revised title is as follows**:（show revised title）

Commonly used verbs are as follows: **checked, edited, proofread, revised, reworded**.

● 英語の質に関するコメントに対しては，修正の必要がない場合は英文校正を受けた旨を伝え，修正の必要がある場合は修正後の文章を示すようにする．

3. Requests for more information
情報の追加を求めるコメントへの対応

Reviewers frequently request more information. Here I provide examples of how to respond.

[**Comment 1**　データの追加を求めるコメント]

Please include the rate of increase.

Response

- <u>The rate of increase has been stated</u> in line 78 of the revised manuscript.

Explanation

The academic verb **stated** is used. Other possible verbs are **included** and **added**. If you use the word **added**, the preposition **to** is needed, **added + to**. (X has been added to Y)

- <u>The rate of increase has been added to</u> line 177 of the revised manuscript.

Examples

- <u>We have included this information in line 177</u> of the revised manuscript.
- <u>This information appears in line 177</u> of the revised manuscript.
- <u>We have added this data to line 177</u> of the revised manuscript.
- <u>This information appears on page 6, line 19</u>.

Please note the following sentence patterns: **in line 17**, **added to line 17**, **on page 17**.

🖉 Key Point

● データを追加したことを述べるには，'stated''included''added to' などの動詞を用いる。

[**Comment 2**　文献の追加を求めるコメント]

Some of the statements on page 6 concerning selection of sites for investigation should be supported by references. There are a lot of relevant references that would help readers such as Edwards 2014.

Response

- **We have cited three references** to support the explanation on page 6. **These are as follows**: Edwards 2014, Stuart 2011 and Yamada 2015.

Explanation

When referring to a reference, the word **cite** is frequently used. Other possible verbs are **add** and **include**.

Examples

- **The following references have been added**: Edwards 2014, Stuart 2011 and Yamaguchi 2015.
- **We included the following references**: Suzuki 2016 and Watanabe 2012.

Short response

- **We have cited** Williams 2015.

🖊 Key Point

● 文献を追加したときは，'cite' 'add' 'include' などを用いる．

[**Comment 3**　説明の追加を求めるコメント]

In the Conclusion, the authors state that the system has several applications. Please briefly describe one application.

Response

- **We have added the following explanation to page 17 of the revised manuscript**. (show revised version)

Explanation

The authors use the expression, **We have added X to Y**. In the examples below, the verbs **given** and **provided** are used.

Examples

- **We have given one example of** a possible application on page 17.
- A brief description of one application **has been provided on page 17**.
- **We have provided** a brief description of an application **on page 17**.

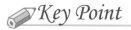
Key Point

● Y の箇所に X の記述を加筆したときは，'We have added X to Y' などの表現を用いて説明する．

[Comment 4　追加のデータ解析を求めるコメント]

Most frequencies were recorded at sites outside urban areas. The authors should carefully discuss their results in terms of location. Is the data from urban, semi-urban and rural areas handled separately? What is the role of the location?

Response

- <u>Additional data analysis was performed to address</u> potential roles of location. <u>The methods used to evaluate and analyze signals have been described</u>. <u>Average rates were calculated</u> for all the sites mentioned. <u>The results are reported in</u> the revised version of Table 3 <u>and explained in the text on page 17</u>.

Explanation

The response is in 4 steps. You will note that the authors do not summarize the reviewer's comment and that sentences are passive.

1. State that additional data analysis was performed and for what reason

- <u>Additional data analysis was performed to address</u> potential roles of location.

2. State the added information

- <u>The methods used to evaluate and analyze signals have been described</u>.

3. State that rates for all sites are provided

- <u>Average rates were calculated for</u> all the sites mentioned.

4. State that results are given in a table and information in the text

- <u>The results are reported in</u> the revised version of Table 3 and <u>explained in the text on page 17</u>.

Examples

1. State that further data analysis was performed

- **We carried out further data analysis to analyze** potential roles of location.

2. State the added information

- **We provided details of ways of evaluating** and analyzing signals.

3. State that rates for all sites are provided

- **From the above analysis, we estimated** the role of location.

4. State that results are given in a table and information in the text

- **We have presented** the results of the above analysis in the revised table, **which is backed up by** a detailed explanation on page 7.

Key Point

- 追加のデータ解析を行った場合は，どのような解析を行ってどのような結果が得られたか，段階を踏んで説明する．

Comment 5　追加の説明を求めるコメント

For the reasons listed above, I think that the underlying mechanism is not adequately described by the authors. This is a serious issue that should be addressed.

Response

- **We note that the reviewer is concerned about** our analysis of the mechanism. **To address this issue, we have conducted** a new series of experiments. **The findings are on** page 17 of the revised manuscript, and **can be summarized as follows:** (show a numbered list of the main findings). **We feel that the new data provides** a good description of the mechanism and how it works. **We trust this answers the concerns raised by the reviewer**.

Explanation

In the above example, the response can be divided into five steps.

1. Refer to the issue raised

- <u>We note that the reviewer is concerned about</u> our analysis of the mechanism.

2. Explain how you have addressed the above problem

- <u>To address this issue, we have conducted</u> a series of experiments.

3. Summarize the results/findings

- <u>The findings are on</u> page 17 of the revised manuscript, and <u>can be summarized as follows</u>: (show a numbered list of the main findings)

4. Explain why the changes to the manuscript are appropriate

- <u>We feel that the new data provides</u> a good description of the mechanism and how it works.

5. Finish the response

- <u>We trust this answers the concerns raised by the reviewer</u>.

Examples

1. Refer to the issue raised

- <u>The reviewer has questioned</u> our analysis of the mechanism.

2. Explain how you have addressed the above problem

- A series of additional experiments <u>have been carried out</u>.

3. Summarize the results/findings

- <u>This is a brief summary of the main findings</u>. (show a numbered list of the main findings)

4. Explain why the changes to the manuscript are appropriate

- <u>We consider that</u> the new data and accompanying information <u>increases our knowledge of</u> the mechanism and how it works.

5. Finish the response

- <u>We hope this answers the points raised by the reviewer</u>.

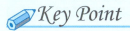
Key Point

- 説明が不十分であることを指摘された場合，必要に応じて追加の実験などを行って対応することもある．
- 追加の実験を行った場合は，どのような実験を行ってどのような結果が得られたか，段階を踏んで説明する．

| Summary | **Requests for more information**
情報の追加を求めるコメントへの対応 |

Frequently used sentence patterns are as follows:

- The rate of increase **has been stated in line 75**.
- **We have included** this information **in line 75**.
- **This information has been included** in line 75.
- **We have added** two references **to** the Introduction.
- **We have provided more information about** sampling procedures.
- **We have given one example of** an application.
- **One example of an application has been given**.
- **We have cited** several additional references.
- **Several additional references have been cited**.

The following verbs are commonly used: **add**, **cite**, **give**, **include**, **provide**, **state**.

- 情報の追加を求めるコメントを受け取り，要請どおりに情報を追加した場合には，'add' 'include' などを用いてそのことを説明する．

4 Clarifying a point
記述を明確にするよう求めるコメントへの対応

Reviewers frequently request that authors improve the clarity of their manuscripts. Here are some model responses.

[**Comment 1**　記述を明確にするよう求めるコメント]

In the Methods section, it is stated that some participants filled out a questionnaire, while others had face-to-face interviews. From the description given, it is difficult to see what the differences were and why you employed two methods of collecting data. An explanation is necessary.

Response

- **The reviewer has commented on** the lack of clarity concerning data collection in the Methods section, page 12, lines 15 ~ 20. **Our point was that** information from the study participants was collected in two ways: by face-to-face interviews and questionnaires. **The reason for this was that** some participants were unable to attend the medical center because of the distance and travel time involved. **We agree that** these two methods differ, **but do not consider** this to be a serious issue. **We note that** Bennett (2014) uses the same methods of collecting data in a study with similar goals. **We have, however, added** several lines to the manuscript explaining why two different methods of collecting information were used. **Additionally, we have cited the paper by Bennet. The revised version is as follows**: (show revised version)

Explanation

The response consists of nine main steps.

1. The authors state the issue raised by the reviewer

- **The reviewer has commented on** the lack of clarity concerning data collection in the Methods section, page 12, lines 15 ~ 20.

2. The authors explain the point they wanted to make

- **Our point was that** information from the study participants was collected in two ways: by face-to-face interviews and questionnaires.

3. The authors give the reason for the point made in 2 above

- **The reason for this was that** some participants were unable to attend the medical center because of the distance and travel time involved.

4. The authors accept the point made by the reviewer

- **We agree that** these two methods differ, (this sentence is continued in example 5 below)

5. The authors comment on the point made by the reviewer

- **but do not consider** this to be a serious issue.

6. The authors give information to support their argument

- **We note that** Bennett (2014) uses the same methods of collecting data in a study with similar goals.

7. The authors state they have added several lines of explanation

- **We have, however, added** several lines to the manuscript explaining why two different methods of collecting information were used.

8. The authors state that a reference has been added

- **Additionally, we have cited** the paper by Bennet.

9. The authors finish their response

- **The revised version is as follows**: (show revised version)

Examples

1. The authors introduce the issue raised by the reviewer

- **The reviewer is concerned about lack of clarity** in the Methods section.

2. The authors explain the point they wanted to make

- **We wanted to say/state/point out that** data was collected in two ways.

3. The authors give the reason

- **This was because** some participants had to travel long distances.

4. The authors accept the point made by the reviewer

- **We accept that** the two methods differ.

5. The authors comment on the point made by the reviewer

- <u>We do not think/consider</u> this a serious issue.

6. The authors give information to support their argument

- <u>We would like to point out that</u> Bennett (2014) uses the same methods of collecting data in a study with similar goals.

7. The authors state they have added several lines of explanation

- <u>We have explained why</u> two different methods of data collection have been used.

8. The authors add a reference

- <u>The paper by Bennett has been cited</u>.

9. The authors finish their response

- <u>The revised version is shown below with the changes in red</u>.

Short response

It is possible to shorten the above 9-step example to just four steps. Here is an example.

- <u>Thank you for your comment. We realize that our original explanation was unclear and have revised it for clarity. The revised version is as follows:</u> (show revised version)

The author accepts the reviewer's comment, but does not attempt to clarify the original point made or justify the changes made.

1. Thank the reviewer
Please note that this step could be omitted and the response started from 2. This would reduce it to three steps.

- <u>Thank you for your comment</u>.

2. Accept the criticism

- <u>We realize that our original explanation was unclear</u>

This sentence is continued in example 3.

3. State that the original version has been revised

- **and have revised it for clarity**.

4. Show the revised version

- **The revised version is as follows:** (show revised version)

Summary

Clarifying a point
記述を明確にするよう求めるコメントへの対応

Frequently used sentence patterns are as follows:

- **The point we wanted to make was that** information from the study participants was collected in two ways.
- **The point we were making was that** information from the study participants was collected in two ways.
- **Our intention was to say/state/point out that** information from the study participants was collected in two ways.
- **What we wanted to say was** that information from the study participants was collected in two ways.
- **We wanted to emphasize that** information from the study participants was collected in two ways.
- **We meant to say that** information from the study participants was collected in two ways.
- 記述の曖昧さを指摘されたときは，'Our point was that' 'The point we wanted to make was that' などの表現を用いて，伝えたいポイントを明確に説明する．
- そのうえで，修正後の文章を 'The revised version is as follows:' の後に続けるとよい．

5 Explaining why you cannot comply with a reviewer's request
なぜ査読者の要請に応えることができないかの説明

Reviewers frequently ask authors to add more information. In some cases, for technical and other reasons, authors will be unable to comply and an explanation will be necessary.

[**Comment 1**　論文の範囲を超えた内容の加筆を求めるコメント]

On page 7, you state that one of the probes can be used to assess levels of inflammation in experimental animals. If possible, a description of how this technique could apply in humans should be added.

Response

- <u>The reviewer has asked for</u> a description of how this technique could apply in humans. <u>Currently, the technique has only been used in experiments on</u> mice, and <u>we are unable to give any information on</u> use in humans. <u>We agree that this is an important area that requires further research, but at present it is beyond the scope of this study. We hope to be able to conduct further studies in the near future that will help us to assess</u> the potential for use in humans.

Explanation

The above response can be divided into five main steps.

1. Summarize the reviewer's request

- <u>The reviewer has asked for</u> a description of how this technique could apply in humans.

2. Explain why you cannot comply with the reviewer's request

- <u>Currently, the technique has only been used in experiments on</u> mice, and <u>we are unable to give any information on</u> use in humans.

3. Agree with the importance of the reviewer's request

- <u>We agree that this is an important area that requires further research,</u> (This sentence is continued in example 4.)

4. State clearly that the request cannot be met

- <u>but at present it is beyond the scope of this study</u>.

Note: Examples 3 and 4 are usually combined. Here is an example.

- **We agree that this is an important area that requires further research, but at present it is beyond the scope of this study.**

5. Refer to future work

- **We hope to be able to conduct further studies in the near future that will** help us to assess the potential for use in humans.

Examples

1. Summarize the reviewer's request

- **The reviewer has requested that** we provide information concerning the use of the technology in humans.
- **The reviewer wants to know** if the technology can be used in humans.
- **The reviewer would like to know** if the technology can be used in humans.
- **The reviewer raised the issue of** use in humans.

2. Explain why you cannot comply with the reviewer's request

- **Since the technique has only been used** in mice, **we cannot comment on** its use in humans.
- The use of this technique in humans **was not one of the goals of this study**.
- **We did not look at** the potential application in humans.

3. Agree with the importance of the reviewer's request

- **We acknowledge the need to** consider the application of this technology in humans, (This sentence is continued in example 4.)
- **We accept that there is a need to** consider the application of this technology in humans,
- **Establishing the potential of this technology in humans is an important goal**,

4. State clearly that the request cannot be met

- **however, it is currently not feasible**.
- **however, we were unable to address** that subject in this research.
- **but, currently it is technically not possible**.

Note: Examples 3 and 4 are frequently combined to form one sentence. Here is an example.

- <u>Establishing the potential of this technology in humans is an important goal, however, it is currently not feasible.</u>

5. Refer to future work

- <u>We are planning to carry out</u> further studies on the probe's potential in humans.
- Potential applications of this technology <u>will be one of the topics of our future research.</u>

🖉 Key Point

● 論文の範囲を超えた内容について加筆するよう求められた場合は，それに応じることができないことを，理由とともに明確に示す．

[**Comment 2** 入手不可能なデータの提示を求めるコメント]

The use of fertilizer in this study should be described, particularly the amount and quality.

Response

- <u>Unfortunately, we could not obtain this information. Farmers involved in this study did not keep records of fertilizer type, amount or grade and, for that reason, it was not included.</u>

Explanation

The reviewer has asked for more detailed information. The authors are unable to provide that data and explain the reason why.

The response is divided into two main steps.

1. State that you cannot comply with the request

- <u>Unfortunately, we could not obtain this information.</u>

2. Explain the reason

- <u>Farmers involved in this study did not keep records of fertilizer type, amount or grade and, for that reason, it was not included.</u>

Examples

1. State that you cannot comply with the request

- <u>We were unable to obtain data on</u> use of fertilizer.
- <u>It was not possible to obtain the data</u>.

2. Explain the reason

- <u>Since some farmers had no records, it was not possible to provide</u> any information.
- <u>Data on the use of fertilizer cannot be provided</u> as farmers had no reliable records.

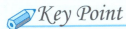
Key Point

● 要請されたデータを用意することができない場合は，その理由を説明する．

Summary — Explaining why you cannot comply with a reviewer's request
なぜ査読者の要請に応えることができないかの説明

When you cannot comply with a reviewer's request, the following five steps can be used.

1. Summarize the reviewers' request

- <u>The reviewer requested that</u> we give a description of how the system can be applied.
- <u>The reviewer wants us to explain</u> how the system can be applied.
- <u>The reviewers have asked for</u> a description of how the system can be applied.

2. State why you cannot comply

- <u>At present, it is technically impossible to</u> give a detailed analysis of future uses.
- <u>We are unable to comment on future uses because</u> it was not one of the aims of this study.
- The use of this technique in humans <u>was not one of the goals of this research</u>.

3. Agree with the importance of the reviewer's comment

- <u>We understand that potential use in humans is an area of interest</u>.
- <u>The reviewer is right to point out</u> the need to consider use in humans.
- <u>We agree that this is an important area,</u> but currently we cannot comment on it.

4. State clearly that the request cannot be met

- <u>Currently for technical reasons, we are unable to comment on</u> potential use in humans.
- <u>At present, potential use in humans is beyond the scope of this study</u>.
- We agree that this is an important area, **but currently we cannot comment on it**.

5. Refer to future work

- <u>We hope to be able to comment on this issue</u> in a future study/after further experiments.
- <u>We hope to be able to conduct studies that will help us to</u> understand the mechanism.
- <u>We are planning to focus on this issue in future research</u>.

Frequently used verbs are as follows:
altered, changed, corrected, deleted, rectified, revised, rewritten, should be.
The verb **read** is used to indicate the revised version. For example: **The revised version reads as follows**: (show revised version)

● 査読者の要請に応えられないときは，その理由をはっきりと説明する必要がある．

Notes on responding to reviewers' comments

10

Grammar choices: We have added vs We added

時制の選択：現在完了形？　過去形？

I was recently asked if there is any difference between the following sentences.
- *We have revised the Introduction.*
- *We revised the Introduction.*

There is no difference in meaning between the two sentences and both are grammatically correct. The main difference is in level of formality. <u>Have revised</u> is slightly more formal than <u>revised</u>.

In **Notes on responding to reviewers' comments 9**, page 98, I discussed the question of how short a response can be and gave examples of one word responses. For example, some authors use <u>revised</u> as a one word response. Below we have three sentences with the same meaning but different grammar and levels of formality.
1. *We have revised the Introduction.*
2. *We revised the Introduction.*
3. *Revised.*

If you are concerned about retaining a degree of formality, example 1 is the best choice. If you are less worried about formality, you can use example 2. If you have a large number of corrections in the Minor comments section, example 3 is useful. Other verbs commonly used in the Minor comments section as one word responses are as follows: <u>added</u>, <u>defined</u>, <u>deleted</u>, <u>fixed</u>, <u>omitted</u>, <u>revised</u>, <u>rewritten</u>.

6 Explaining why you do not want to make a suggested change
なぜ変更の提案に応じないかの説明

In most cases, authors will need to comply with requests from editors and reviewers. There will, however, be times when authors cannot agree with proposed changes and careful wording of the response is necessary. Here are some model responses to help you handle this situation.

Comment 1　図の変更を求めるコメント

In Figs. 2 and 3, I feel the authors should superimpose dose distribution on both figures.

Response

- <u>The reviewer has asked that</u> we superimpose dose distribution on Figures 2 and 3. <u>We consider that as they stand</u> Figures 2 and 3 give a fast visual demonstration of dosage. <u>We think that</u> superimposing them would have a negative effect on the visual impact of the figure. <u>For this reason, we would like to keep</u> the figures as they are.

Explanation

This response has four steps.

1. Summarize the reviewer's request

- <u>The reviewer has asked that</u> we superimpose dose distribution on Figures 2 and 3.

2. Explain why you think no change is necessary

- <u>We consider that as they stand</u> Figures 2 and 3 give a fast visual demonstration of dosage.

3. State why you cannot agree with the reviewer's request

- <u>We think that superimposing them would have a negative effect on</u> the visual impact of the figure.

4. Refer to the reason given in 3. and state that you cannot comply with the request

- <u>For this reason, we would like to keep</u> the figures as they are.

Examples

1. Summarize the reviewer's request

- <u>The reviewer has requested that</u> we superimpose dose distribution on Figures 2 and 3.
- <u>The reviewer wants us/would like us</u> to superimpose dose distribution on Figures 2 and 3.
- <u>The reviewer has suggested superimposing</u> dose distribution on Figures 2 and 3.

2. Explain why you think no change is necessary

- <u>In our opinion</u>, Figures 2 and 3 give a fast visual demonstration of dosage.

3. State why you cannot agree with the reviewer's request

- <u>We feel that superimposing them would have a negative effect on</u> the visual impact of the figure.
- <u>We think that superimposing them would have a negative effect on</u> the visual impact of the figure.

4. Refer to the reason given in 3. and state that you cannot comply with the request

- <u>For the above reason, we would prefer not to change</u> the figures.
- <u>For this reason/For these reasons, we are reluctant to</u> make the suggested changes.
- <u>For this reason/For these reasons, we would prefer not to</u> make the suggested changes.
- <u>Taking into account the above points, we would prefer not to</u> make the suggested changes.

🖉 Key Point

● 査読者からの提案に対して，自分の考えを説明する際は，'We consider that' や 'In our opinion' を用いる．

Comment 2　研究対象者の変更を求めるコメント

I am concerned about the fact that all subjects in the study were institutionalized adults. It is necessary to verify their degree of general fitness and mobility at the outset. It may also be necessary to exclude those at the lowest range of mobility. These are serious issues requiring further explanation and justification.

Response

- <u>The aim of this study was to examine</u> the hypothesis that structured exercise programs for aged people living in institutions reduce the number of falls. <u>As previous studies have reported, this kind of study is appropriate for</u> institutionalized adults and, <u>therefore, we consider that verification of general fitness is not essential for this study</u>. However, <u>we agree that more patient information</u> particularly concerning mobility, previous experience of similar programs, and history of falls <u>would help to validate the results</u>. <u>Accordingly, we have added background information on</u> the patients. <u>The following description has been added</u> to the manuscript.（show revised version）

Explanation

The response can be divided into six main steps as follows:

1. Restate the aim of the study

- <u>The aim of this study was to examine the hypothesis that</u> structured exercise programs for aged people living in institutions reduce the number of falls.

2. State known information/refer to previous studies

- <u>As previous studies have reported, this kind of study is appropriate for institutionalized adults and,</u>（This sentence is continued in example 3.）

3. Give a reason why you are not accepting the reviewer's suggestion

- <u>therefore, we consider that verification of general fitness is not essential for this study</u>.

4. Compromise

- **However, we agree that** more patient information particularly concerning mobility, previous experience of similar programs, and history of falls **would help to validate the results**.

5. Add information

- **Accordingly, we have added background information on** the patients.

6. Show revised version

- **The following description has been added to** the manuscript. (show revised version)

Examples

1. Restate the aim of the study

- **In this study, we wanted to examine the hypothesis that** structured exercise programs for aged people living in institutions reduce the number of falls.

2. State known information/refer to previous studies

- **It is known that** this kind of study is appropriate for institutionalized adults.

3. Give a reason why you are not accepting the reviewer's suggestion

- **For that reason**, we consider verification of general levels of fitness is not essential.

4. Compromise

- **We accept that** more patient information particularly concerning mobility and history of falls would add validity to the study.

5. Add information

- **Relevant background information on patients has been included**.

6. Show revised version

- **This reads as follows**: (show revised version)

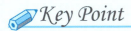

Key Point

- 研究対象を広げるべきだという指摘に対しては，論文の目的を説明することで対処する．

Comment 3　記述の変更を求めるコメント

On page 17, line 21, the authors state that 'patients involved in 3-week therapy trials showed improvement in mobility, balance and cognitive tasks'. There is no data presented in the manuscript to support the above statement, and the authors do not provide any specific references or refer to the literature. These issues should be addressed.

Response

- <u>The reviewer has raised concerns regarding</u> supporting data for the statement on page 17, line 21. **<u>While we accept the reviewer's concerns, we would like to keep this sentence, because we believe that</u>** it gives a good overall picture of the benefits of the therapy program. Tests on mobility, balance and cognitive ability were carried out during the study, but the results were not included in the original manuscript. **<u>We have added a Table showing those results. In addition, we have added</u>** one reference as follows: Williams 2015. **<u>The approach we have adopted</u>**, as well as our results, **<u>are generally in line with those of Williams</u>**. **<u>We hope that this explanation and the addition of a reference meet with the approval of the reviewer</u>**.

Explanation

This response has seven steps.

1. Summarize the reviewer's comment and the issue

- <u>The reviewer has raised concerns regarding</u> supporting data for the statement on page 17, line 21.

2. State that you want to retain the sentence

- <u>While we accept the reviewer's concerns, we would like to keep this sentence</u>, (This sentence is continued in example 3.)

3. Give a reason why you want to retain the sentence

- <u>because we believe that</u> it gives a good overall picture of the benefits of the therapy program.

4. State that you have added a Table showing results

- <u>We have added a Table showing those results</u>.

5. State that you have added a reference

- **In addition, we have added one reference as follows**: Williams 2015.

6. Explain how the reference is relevant

- **The approach we have adopted**, as well as our results, **are generally in line with those of Williams**.

7. Finish your response

- **We hope that this explanation and the addition of a reference meet with the approval of the reviewer**.

Examples

1. Summarize the reviewer's comment and the issue

- **The reviewer is concerned about** supporting data for the statement on page 17, line 21.

2. State that you want to retain the sentence

- **We agree that this a potential issue, but we are reluctant to change the text as it provides** a concise and accurate description of the results.

3. Give a reason why you want to retain the sentence

- **Since the description of the results provides a concise and accurate picture, we would prefer to** leave it as it is.

4. State that you have added a Table showing results

- **A Table showing the results has been added**.

5. State that you have added a reference

- **To overcome this issue, we have cited** one reference as follows: Williams 2015.

6. Explain how the reference is relevant

- **Our approach/methods are largely the same as those adopted by Stuart 2016**.

7. Finish your response

- **We hope that the above responses meet with the approval of** the editors and reviewers.

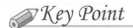
Key Point

● 査読者の指摘を認めつつも変更は行わない場合には，'While we accept the reviewer's concerns, we would like to 〜 , because 〜 .' を用いる．

Summary: Explaining why you do not want to make a suggested change
なぜ変更の提案に応じないのかの説明

1. Summarize the reviewers' request

- <u>The reviewer has asked/requested</u> that we present the information on page 7 in the form of a table.
- <u>The reviewer wants/would like</u> us to present the information on page 7 in the form of a table.
- <u>The reviewer has suggested</u> that we present the information on page 7 in the form of a table.

2. State why you think no change is necessary

- <u>We consider that</u> there is too much detailed information to be presented in a Table.
- <u>In our opinion</u>, there is too much detailed information to be presented in a Table.

3. State why you cannot agree with the reviewer's request

- <u>We think that</u> explaining the details in the text is better for readers.
- <u>We feel that</u> explaining the details in the text is better for readers.

4. State that for the above reason you cannot comply

- <u>For this reason</u>, we would prefer not to include the information in a Table.
- <u>For the above reasons</u>, we would prefer not to include the information in a Table.
- <u>Taking into account the above points</u>, we would prefer not to include the information in a Table.

● 査読者が提案してきた変更を行いたくない場合には，'We consider that' などを用いて自分の考えを説明したうえで，提案に従うことができないことを述べればよい．

7 Responding to critical comments
批判的なコメントへの対応

In this section, I look at how to respond to critical comments.

[**Comment 1**　用語に関する批判的コメント]

I note that the word handicapped is used throughout the manuscript. This term has been unacceptable in the field for several years.

Response
- **We agree that** the term handicapped **is unacceptable and have changed it to** physically challenged.

Explanation
This criticism is mild and only involves the need to change some terminology. In this case, the author accepts the criticism and replies with the following phrase.

- **We agree that** the term handicapped **is unacceptable**.

Other possible words for **unacceptable** are as follows:
incorrect, vague, an error, an issue.

Examples
- **The word handicapped has been changed to** physically challenged throughout the manuscript.
- **We have changed the word handicapped to** physically challenged.
- The word handicapped **has been deleted from the manuscript**.

✏ Key Point
- 不適切な用語の使用を指摘されたときは，'unacceptable' 'incorrect' などの表現を用いて非を認め，別の用語に変更する．

[**Comment 2**　図と文章の食い違いに関する批判的コメント]

The authors state that performance improves steadily. However, Figure 3 shows that performance is intermittent at times. This is a serious inconsistency that should be addressed.

Response

- **We accept that** the phrase 'performance improves steadily' does not match the data shown in Fig. 3. **Accordingly, we have deleted** the word 'steadily' and **described performance in greater detail**. **The revised version is as follows**: (show revised version)

Explanation

This response has three steps.

1. Accept the criticism

- **We accept that** the phrase 'performance improves steadily' does not match the data shown in Fig. 3.

2. Explain the action taken

- **Accordingly, we have deleted** the word 'steadily' and **described performance in greater detail**.

3. Show the revised version

- **The revised version is as follows**: (show revised version)

Examples

1. Accept the criticism

- **The reviewer is right to point out that** the phrase 'performance improves steadily' does not match the data.
- **We agree that** the phrase 'performance improves steadily' is an issue.
- **It is correct to say that** there is a discrepancy between the data in Fig 3 and our descriptions.

2. Explain the action taken

- **We have changed/deleted** the word 'steadily'.
- **We have revised this section**.
- **We have moved this sentence to** the Discussion section.

3. Show the revised version

- **The revised sentence is/sentences are shown in the text in red**.
- **Changes are shown in the text in red**.

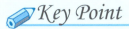
Key Point

- 図表中のデータを本文中で正しく説明できていないことを指摘された場合は，本文を修正する．
- 査読者の指摘を受け入れるときは 'We accept that' や 'We agree that' を用いる．

Comment 3　記述の分かりづらさに関する批判的コメント

On page 17, the authors give information on the subjects. I find this confusing, particularly the explanation concerning the age distribution of subjects.

Response

- <u>The reviewer is concerned about</u> the lack of clarity in our description of the age distribution of the subjects. <u>The reviewer is correct, and we appreciate the chance to make ourselves clearer</u>. <u>We have revised the paper as follows</u>: (show revised version)

Explanation

This response is in three steps.

1. Summarize the problem
The authors briefly summarize the problem raised by the reviewer.

- <u>The reviewer is concerned about</u> the lack of clarity in our description of the age distribution of the subjects.

2. Agree with the reviewer
The authors agree with the point made by the reviewer.

- <u>The reviewer is correct, and we appreciate the chance to make ourselves clearer</u>.

3. State the revision
The authors state the revision.

- <u>We have revised the paper as follows</u>: (show revised version)

Examples

1. Summarize the problem

- **The reviewer pointed out/has pointed out** the lack of clarity in our description of the age distribution of the study subjects.
- **The reviewer is/was concerned about** discrepancies in the statistical analysis.
- **The reviewer raised the issue of** discrepancies in the statistical analysis.

2. Agree with the reviewer

- **We take the reviewer's point about** our description of the age distribution of the subjects.
- **We accept the reviewer's point concerning** our description of the age distribution of the subjects.
- **We agree with the reviewer's point relating to** our description of the age distribution of the subjects.

3. State the revision

- **We have revised the paper as follows**: (show revised version)
- **We have rewritten this sentence as follows**: (show revised version)

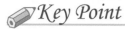Key Point

● 記述が分かりづらいというコメントを受け取った場合は、より簡明な文章に修正する。

Comment 4　記述の妥当性に関する批判的コメント

The authors state the onset of the disease in males is in early middle age, but I am not convinced this is correct. A number of studies have reported men in their early 20s showing signs of the disease. This should be stated.

Response

- **Thank you for your comment concerning** onset of the disease. Although the vast majority of cases reported in the literature are in early middle age, **we accept your point that** a number of cases have recently been reported of men in their early 20's showing signs of the disease. **We have revised this section to reflect this fact. The revised version is shown below.** (show revised version)

Explanation
This response is in four steps.

1. Thanking the reviewer
- <u>Thank you for your comment concerning</u> onset of the disease.

2. Accepting the suggested revision
- <u>We accept your point that</u> a number of cases have recently been reported of men in their early 20's showing signs of the disease.

3. Explaining the change
- <u>We have revised the section to reflect this fact</u>.

4. Showing the revised version
- <u>The revised version is shown below</u>. (show revised version)

Examples

1. Thanking the reviewer
- <u>Thank you for your comment about/on</u> the age of onset.

2. Accepting the suggested revision
- <u>We agree that</u> some cases of men in their early 20's showing signs of the disease have been reported.
- <u>We take your point that</u> some cases of men in their early 20's showing signs of the disease have been reported.

3. Explaining the change
- <u>We have included</u> this information along with the relevant references.
- <u>We have added</u> the relevant information and references to this section.
- <u>We have revised the section</u> to include this data.

4. Showing the revised version
- <u>The revised version is shown below</u>. (show revised version)
- <u>The revised version is as follows</u>. (show revised version)

Short response

- <u>We have revised the text according to the reviewer's comments</u>. <u>It is now as follows</u>: (show revised version)
- <u>We have revised this section to reflect the reviewer's comment concerning age of onset</u>. <u>The revised version is as follows</u>: (show revised version)

✏️ Key Point

● 記述が正確さに欠けていることを指摘された場合は，査読者への感謝を述べたうえで，文章を修正する．

Summary | **Responding to critical comments**
批判的なコメントへの対応

This is a summary of how to respond to critical comments. All of the responses in this section show cases where **the authors accept the criticism and make the necessary changes according to the reviewers' comments.**

1. Thank the reviewer

- <u>Thank you for your comments concerning/about/on</u> (topic).

2. Accept the reviewer's comment

- <u>We accept/agree that</u> some cases of men in their early 20's showing signs of the disease have been reported.
- <u>We take your point that</u> some cases of men in their early 20's showing signs of the disease have been reported.

3. Explain how you have handled the criticism

- <u>We have revised this section by</u> adding more data.
- <u>We have added some more data to this section</u>.

4. Show revised version

- <u>The revised version is shown below</u>. (show revised version)

● 批判的なコメントを受け取り，その批判を受け入れる場合には，はじめに査読者の指摘に感謝し，そのうえでどのように修正したかを説明するとよい．

Part 6
Common errors

In this part, I introduce common errors in responses to reviewers' comments. Errors are divided into the following categories:

(1) **grammar** (2) **vocabulary** (3) **expressions**.

× = Error
○ = Revised version
E = Explanation

1. Grammar errors

✗ Reviewer 1 recommended **us** to add more experimental results.

○ Reviewer 1 **recommended that we add** more experimental results.

○ Reviewer 1 **recommended adding** more experimental results.

E It is not correct to follow the verb **recommend** with 'us'. The correct grammatical patterns are: recommend + that + verb, recommend + verb + ing.

✗ We thank **reviewers for careful** reading our manuscript.

○ We thank **the** reviewers for **carefully** reading our manuscript.

○ We **wish to** thank **the** reviewers for **carefully** reading our manuscript.

○ **We would like to thank the reviewers** for **carefully** reading our manuscript.

E The expression **we thank reviewers** is incorrect. A definite article is necessary before the word reviewers, thank **the** reviewers. It is also possible to use the following expressions: **we wish to thank the reviewers**, **we would like to thank the reviewers**. The word '**careful**' should be changed to carefully.

✗ **To make the sense clearly,** we have changed the sentence as follows:

○ **To improve clarity,** we have changed the sentence as follows: (show revised version)

○ **To make the meaning clearer,** we have changed the sentence as follows: (show revised version)

E The expression **to make the sense clearly** is incorrect. Better expressions are as follows: **to improve clarity**, **to make the meaning clearer**, **to make it easier to understand**. The shortest reply is. **We have changed the sentence as follows:** (show revised version)

132   Part 6 Common errors

✗	<u>According to the reviewer's comments,</u> we have revised the sentence.
○	**Based on the reviewer's comments,** we have revised the sentence.
○	**In line with the reviewer's comments,** we have revised the sentence.
E	According to the reviewer's comments is overused by Japanese authors and incorrect in this context. **Based on the reviewer's comments** or **in line with the reviewer's comments** are better. It should be remembered, however, that these expressions should not be used in every response. In this case, the shortest response is as follows: **We have revised the sentence**.
✗	The reviewer is correct **by** pointing out the statistical error.
○	The reviewer is correct **to point out/in pointing** out the statistical error.
E	The sentence structure should be **correct to point out**, **correct in pointing out**.
✗	<u>Reviewer</u> is right.
○	**The reviewer** is right.
E	Before the word **reviewer,** the definite article **the** is required. The word **correct** can also be used in this example. **The reviewer is correct to point out/in pointing out** that the statistical analysis is incorrect.

✗	<u>Majority</u> of data is derived from different locations.
○	**<u>The majority of</u>** data is derived from different locations.
○	**<u>Most of the</u>** data is derived from different locations.
○	**<u>Most</u>** data is derived from different locations.
○	**<u>Almost all of the</u>** data is derived from different locations.
E	Before the word **majority,** the definite article **<u>the</u>** is needed. **<u>The majority of</u>** (X). Other similar patterns are as follows: **<u>most of the data</u>**, **<u>most data</u>**, **<u>almost all of the data</u>**, **<u>almost all data</u>**. Please note that <u>almost data</u> is incorrect. The correct pattern is **<u>almost all data</u>**, **<u>almost all of the data</u>**.
✗	The solution <u>for</u> this problem is now being <u>searched</u>.
○	We are now **<u>looking for</u>** a solution **<u>to</u>** this problem.
○	We are now **<u>searching for</u>** a solution **<u>to</u>** this problem.
○	We are now **<u>trying to find</u>** a solution **<u>to</u>** this problem.
E	It is better to change the word order of the sentence and start with **<u>we</u>**. Please note that the preposition following the word solution is **<u>to</u>**. The verbs **<u>looking for</u>**, **<u>searching for</u>** and **<u>trying to find</u>** can be used.

X	We did not **succeed to obtain** any reliable data.
O	We did not **succeed in obtaining any** reliable data.
O	**We did not manage to obtain** any reliable data.
O	**We were unable to obtain** any reliable data.
O	We **did not obtain** any reliable data.
E	The simplest way of expressing this is with the following sentences. **We did not obtain any reliable data**. **No reliable data was found/obtained**. The grammar pattern for the word **succeed** is as follows: **succeed in obtaining**.
X	These species **are coexist** in the same environment.
O	These species **coexist/are coexisting** in the same environment.
E	The word **coexist** is a verb and should not be preceded by the verb are unless the sentence is in the present continuous tense.
X	The reviewers' comments have helped us to improve **readability** of the manuscript.
O	The reviewers' comments have helped us to improve **the readability** of the manuscript.
O	**The readability of the manuscript has been improved** as a result of the reviewers' comments.
E	The word **readability** requires a definite article. Other grammatically similar examples are as follows: improve **the** organization/improve **the** structure.

✗	Our **response for** the first reviewer is as follows.
○	Our **responses to** the first reviewer are as follows. (show a numbered list of responses)
○	Below please find our **responses to** the first reviewer's comments. (show a numbered list of responses)
E	The noun **response** should be followed by the word **to** and would generally be plural (**responses**). This sentence is usually used at the beginning of a list of responses to reviewers' comments.

✗	This point is related to **the** comment 1.
○	This point is related **to comment 1**.
E	It is not necessary to have a definite article when a number is given after the word comment. However, **The first comment** is correct.

✗	Ratios are indicated by red **circle**.
○	Ratios are indicated by red **circles**.
○	Ratios are **represented/shown by red circles.**
○	**Red circles represent/show ratios.**
E	In most cases, when referring to circles, arrows or triangles that appear in figures, you will **use the plural form** (circles) as there will probably be more than one in the figure. In cases where there is only one circle, the sentence would be as follows: **The ratio is indicated by a red circle.** **A red circle indicates the ratio**.

✗	We agree that there <u>was a</u> repetition in the Introduction.
○	We agree that there is **some** repetition in the Introduction.
○	We agree that there is **a lot of** repetition in the Introduction.
○	We agree that there is **repetition** in the Introduction.
○	We agree that **repetition** is an issue in the Introduction.
E	The word **repetition** is uncountable and cannot be used with 'a' as in the above incorrect sentence. You can use **some** or **a lot of** before the word repetition. For example, There is **some/a lot of repetition** in the Discussion section. In examples 3 and 4, the word repetition is used without 'some' or 'a lot of'.

✗	We did not show <u>a</u> direct evidence.
○	We did not show **any** direct evidence.
○	We did not show **direct evidence**.
○	**Direct evidence** has not been shown.
E	The word **evidence** is uncountable. It is not possible to say, This is **an evidence**. In a negative sentence, the grammar pattern is as follows: **We did not show any direct evidence**.

✗	<u>We added</u>, 'further sites were investigated'.
○	We added **the phrase**, 'further sites were investigated'.
○	We added **the sentence**, 'There was no significant impact' to line 7 of the Discussion.
○	We added **the word** 'significant' to line 73 of the text.
E	After the word **added**, you need **word**, **phrase**, or **sentence**.

✗	We do not agree with this comment <u>by several following</u> reasons.
○	We do not agree with this comment **for the following** reasons. (show a list of reasons)
E	The preposition used with the word reasons is **for**. (**For this reason**, **For these reasons**, **For the above reason**, **For the following reasons**).

✗	Figure 6 shows an increase of 10 percent. This <u>was</u> a mistake.
○	Figure 6 shows an increase of 10 percent. This **is** a mistake.
E	The present tense should be used in this case.

✗	<u>A</u> paper by Williams (2009) has been cited in the text
○	**The** paper by Williams (2009) has been cited in the text.
○	**<u>We have cited Williams (2009) in the text</u>**.
E	Since this sentence refers to a specific paper and the year of publication is given, the definite article is required. **The paper** by Williams (2009) has been cited in the text.

✗ Language revision **has been done** by a native speaker.

○ This paper **has been revised by a native speaker of English**.

○ **The manuscript has been revised/proofread/checked by a native speaker of English**.

E The expression **has been done** is correct, but more formally it would be expressed as follows: **has been revised**. I have also changed the expression **language revision** to **this paper**. **The manuscript**, **the paper** or **the MS** (abbreviation for the word manuscript) are also possible. Similar words to revised are **checked** and **proofread**.

✗ This reference has been added **in** the Introduction.

○ This reference has been added **to** the Introduction.

○ The following reference has been added **to** the Introduction.

E The correct preposition following the verb **add** is **to**.

✗ Further laboratory studies **should be needed** to verify the effects of this treatment.

○ Further laboratory studies **are needed/necessary/required** to verify the effects of this treatment.

○ Further laboratory studies **should be carried out/should be performed** to verify the effects of this treatment.

E The phrase **should be needed** is incorrect. It should be **are needed/necessary/required**. However, grammatically similar patterns such as **should be carried out** and **should be performed** are possible and can be used here. For example, **Further laboratory studies should be carried out/should be performed**.

✗	We **must add** the description of the Dunnett test, since the description **was missing**.
○	In the original manuscript, **we failed to describe why we used the Dunnett test. This information has now been added to the manuscript**.
E	In this example, the author admits that some necessary information was omitted from the original manuscript. The best way of doing this is to use the expressions: **we failed to describe**, **we omitted to describe**, **we did not describe/include**. Also, please note the useful expressions, **in the original manuscript/in the previous version of this paper**.
✗	I **was** submitting **herewith** a manuscript entitled, (title of the paper).
○	I **am** submitting a manuscript entitled, (title of the paper).
○	**Please find attached** our paper entitled, (title of the paper).
E	The use of the past tense **was** is incorrect. The term **herewith** has been deleted because it is too formal and normally associated with legal documents. Responses to reviewers' comments should use academic English, but there is no advantage in using extremely formal English such as **herewith**.
✗	The reviewer **concerns** about reliability.
○	The reviewer **is concerned about** reliability.
○	The reviewer **expressed concerns about** reliability.
○	**The reviewer thinks that reliability is an issue**.
E	The correct structure for the word **concern** is **be concerned about**. In the following sentence, concern is used as a noun. **The reviewer expressed concerns about reliability**.

✗	**Modified points were described** in red
○	**Changes are shown in the manuscript** in red.
○	**Revisions to the manuscript are indicated** in red.
○	**Changes to/in the manuscript are** in red.
○	**Changes are in red**.
E	The expression **modified points** is incorrect. It should be **changes**, **revisions** or **alterations**. There is also a problem with the expression **were described**. The present tense **are** is correct, not the past tense **were**. The verb **described** should be **shown** or **indicated**. Please note that both of the following are possible: Changes **to** the manuscript/Changes in the manuscript. The shortest possible response is as follows: **Changes are in red**.
✗	The reviewer **told us to remove Table 2**.
○	The reviewer **suggested that we delete Table 2**.
○	The reviewer **asked that we delete Table 2**.
○	The reviewer **asked us to delete Table 2**.
○	The reviewer **requested that we delete Table 2**.
E	The expression **told us to remove** is not correct in this situation, as it is too informal and conversational. It is better to use **suggested**, **asked**, **requested**. The word **delete** is used more frequently than remove.

✗	**It was added the Figure for clarity.**
○	**To improve clarity, a Figure has been added.**
○	**We have added a Figure to improve clarity.**
E	The sentence structure is incorrect. It is better to start the sentence with **to improve clarity** or **we have added a Figure**.
✗	We decided to **increase following reference** and **sentence in methods**.
○	We have added **the following references and sentences to the Methods section**.
○	**The following references and sentences have been added to the Methods section.**
○	**We have added several references and sentences to the Methods section.**
○	**Several references and sentences have been added to the Methods section.**
E	Before the word **following**, you need the definite article **the**. Also **reference** and **sentence** should be in the plural form **references** and **sentences**. **Methods** should be changed to **the Methods section**.
✗	We have added some sentences **in Introduction for clarity of readers**.
○	**To improve clarity,** we have added **several sentences to the Introduction**.
○	**To help readers,** we have added **several sentences to the Introduction**.
E	The expression **in Introduction for clarity of readers** is not correct and has been changed to **to the Introduction**. The expression **to help readers** has been added at the start of the sentence. The following expressions are also possible: **for clarity and** to **improve clarity**.

✗	We added <u>this</u> sentence.
○	We added **the following sentence**. (show the added sentence)
○	**The following sentence has been added**. (show the added sentence)
E	The sentence **'We added X'** is correct and can be used in replies to reviewers' comments. However, **this sentence** should be changed to **the following sentence**. It is more formal and academic to use **the passive form 'X has been added'**.

✗	<u>Base</u> on your comments, the description on page 7 has been <u>excluded</u> from the manuscript.
○	**Based** on the reviewer's comments, the description on page 7 has been **deleted**.
○	**We have deleted the description on page 7**.
○	**The description on page 7 has been deleted**.
○	**The description on page 7 has been omitted**.
○	**The description on page 7 has been removed**.
E	The expression **base on** is grammatically incorrect. It should be **based on**. The word **excluded** is incorrect and should be changed to **deleted**, **omitted** or **removed**. The word **deleted** is used most frequently. Although I have included the phrase **based on the reviewer's comments** in the revised sentence, it could be deleted. The shortest response is the best. **We have deleted the description on page 7**.

✗	We added some basic data <u>in the Table 1</u> and the sampling locations <u>were also added in the</u> Section 2.1.
○	We added some basic data **to Table 1 and sampling locations to Section 2.1**.
E	In the revised sentence, the word **added** is only used once. It is not necessary to have the definite article **the** before Table 1 or Section 2.1. The correct preposition to use with added is **to**. For example **X is added to Y**. The expression, <u>were also added</u>, is redundant and has been deleted from the revised sentence.

✗	Please <u>refer</u> our detailed answer to comments 16 and 17.
○	Please **refer to** our detailed answer to comments 16 and 17.
E	The preposition used with refer is **to**. For example, **please refer to**.

✗	Because we **did** not have any information **of** rates of decay, we cannot comment on this.
○	**Since** we **do** not have any information **on** rates of decay, we cannot comment on this.
○	**We do not have any information on rates of decay**.
E	This sentence should be in the present tense. The verb **did** should be **do**. The expression **information of rates of decay** should be **information on rates of decay** or **information concerning rates of decay**. The sentence can start with either **since** or **because**.

✗	We **agreed** that there **was** too much repetition in the Introduction and have deleted several sentences.
○	We **agree** that there **is** too much repetition in the Introduction and have deleted several sentences.
○	**We agree that repetition is an issue** and have deleted several sentences in the Introduction.
○	**We accept that there is** too much repetition in the Introduction.
○	**We have deleted several sentences in the Introduction. Changes are in red**.
○	**We have reduced the Introduction in length by 15 lines**.
E	The sentence has the same problem as the above example. The **present tense** is better than the **past tense**. The expression **we agree that** can be omitted as shown in the last example sentence. Again, the shortest response is probably the best. **We have deleted several sentences in the Introduction**.
✗	The site locations **were** shown in the revised Table.
○	The site locations **are** shown in the revised Table.
○	The site locations **now appear** in the revised Table.
○	The revised Table now **has** the site locations.
E	Again, this is a problem of tense. **Were** should be **are**.

6.1 Grammar errors

✗	The **differences of** the rate of increase have been stated.
○	**The differences in** the rate of increase have been stated.
○	**Differences in** the rate of increase have been stated.
○	**Differences in** the rate of increase **have been included**.
E	The problem here is the preposition after the word **differences**. The correct preposition is **in**. In the second and third examples, the definite article **the** before the word differences has been omitted.
✗	We added some more information **in the caption of Figure 2**.
○	We added some more information **to the Figure 2 caption**.
○	We added some more information **to the caption in Figure 2**.
○	We have reworded **the Figure 2 caption**.
○	**The Figure 2 caption** has been changed.
E	There are two points here. Since the word **added** is used, the preposition should be to. The sentence structure **the caption of Figure 2** should be **the Figure 2 caption** or **the caption in Figure 2**.
✗	**Response for the first review.**
○	**Responses to Reviewer 1**
E	When this sentence is used as **a title at the top of a page of responses**, a period is not necessary. As you will see, the word **response** has been changed to responses. Also the expression, **for the first review** has been changed to to **Reviewer 1**.

✗	We **did** not have any data **of** survival rates.
○	We **do** not have any data **on** survival rates.
○	**We do not have any survival rate data**.
E	This sentence should be in the present tense. Notice that the preposition after data is **on**. The expression data **of** survival rates is not correct. The word **concerning** could also be used. For example: We do not have any **data concerning** survival rates.
✗	The reviewers' comments have been carefully considered and **were** incorporated in the paper.
○	The reviewers' comments have been carefully considered and **incorporated** in the revised manuscript.
E	In the first part of the sentence, the expression **have been carefully considered** is used. In the second part, **were incorporated** is used. To have similar grammatical structures in the same sentence, **were incorporated** should be changed to **have been incorporated**. To avoid repetition **have been incorporated** has been changed to **incorporated**.
✗	We changed the word handicapped **into** physically challenged.
○	The word handicapped **has been changed to** physically challenged.
E	The preposition **into** is incorrect. **Changed into** means to **become something else**. In this case, the correct grammar is **X has been changed to Y**.

✗	<u>Mistakes in reference list</u> have been corrected.
◯	We have corrected the mistakes **in the references**.
◯	**Mistakes in the references** have been corrected.
◯	We have corrected the mistakes **in the list of references**.
E	Both **the references** and **the list of references** can be used.

✗	Due to the **difficulty to collect** a large number of samples, further analysis was not possible.
◯	Due to the **difficulty of collecting** a large number of samples, further analysis was not possible.
◯	Since we had **difficulty in collecting** a large number of samples, further analysis was not possible.
◯	Since it was **difficult to collect** a large number of samples, further analysis was not possible.
E	The pattern **difficulty to collect** is grammatically incorrect. However, **difficult to collect** is correct.

✗	This data will promote further **researches** on biodegradable polymers.
◯	This data will promote further **research** on biodegradable polymers.
E	The word research is usually treated as a collective noun. Although the word **researches** can be found in some dictionaries, the frequency is much lower than that of **research**. Over time, the usage has changed from **researches** to **research**.

✗	We have made significant changes **on** the Conclusion.
○	We have made significant changes **to** the Conclusion.
○	We have made significant changes **in** the Conclusion.
○	The Conclusion **has been changed significantly**.
E	The correct preposition to use with the verb **change** is **to**.

✗	**Thanks for the advices**.
○	**Thank you for the advice**.
○	**We appreciate the advice**.
○	**Thank you for the useful comments and suggestions**.
E	The expression **thanks for** is rather informal and should be **thank you for**. The word advice is usually treated as a collective noun and for that reason **advices** is incorrect.

✗	We believe this manuscript is appropriate for publication **by** the journal of Oral Science.
○	We believe this manuscript is appropriate for publication **in** the Journal of Oral Science.
E	The correct structure is **appropriate for publication in** (journal name). The preposition **by** is used when referring to a publishing company. For example, **This book was published by Oxford University Press**.

6.1 Grammar errors   149

2. Vocabulary

In this section, I introduce vocabulary errors.

✗	We **quoted** the article **of** Yamada 2015.
◯	We **cited** the article **by** Yamada 2015.
◯	**We cited Yamada 2015.**
◯	**Yamada 2015 has been cited.**
E	There are two problems here. The verb **quoted** means that you have included several lines exactly as they appear in the article by Yamada. **Cite** means to refer to something as an example to support an argument. The expression **the article of Yamada** is incorrect. Instead of the word **of**, it is better to use **by**.
✗	As **suggested**, there **was** an error in the figure legend.
◯	As **pointed out**, there **is** an error in the figure legend. This has been corrected.
◯	**The error in the figure legend has been corrected.**
E	The verb suggest is incorrect because the reviewer is not suggesting anything here. The reviewer **has pointed out** an error. Instead of the past tense **was**, the present tense **is** should be used.
✗	We thank the reviewers for their **fruitful** comments.
◯	We thank the reviewers for their **useful** comments and suggestions.
E	The word **fruitful** is too formal and somewhat dated. At the beginning of the sentence, you can use either **we thank** or **we wish to thank**.

✗	We **remained** the term 'biodegradability'.
○	We **have retained** the term' biodegradability'.
○	**We wish to retain the expression** 'rises in line with duration'.
○	**We have kept the word/term/expression/sentence** (+ example).
E	**Remained** is incorrect. It is possible to use **retain** or **keep** as in the above examples. The following are commonly used in this context: **word**, **term**, **expression**, **sentence**.

✗	The term biocompatibility is **inadequate**.
○	The term biocompatibility is **incorrect**.
○	The term biocompatibility is a **mistake**.
○	**We have deleted the term biocompatibility**.
E	The word **inadequate** is not correct because it gives no concrete information on what is wrong. Other possible words are **incorrect**, **wrong**, **vague** or **misleading**.

✗	We have **reconstructed** the Discussion section.
○	We have **restructured** the Discussion section.
○	We have **reorganized** the Discussion section.
E	The word **reconstruct** means to rebuild something that is physical, and should not be used in this context. Better choices are **restructured**, **reorganized** and **rewritten**.

✗	The degree of improvement is **trivial**.
O	The degree of improvement is **insignificant**.
O	The degree of improvement is **not significant**.
O	The degree of improvement is **negligible**.
E	The word **trivial** means unimportant or of little value and in this context is incorrect. It is better to use the following: **insignificant**, **not significant**, **negligible** or **too small**.

✗	The term appended has been **erased** from the manuscript.
O	The term appended has been **deleted** from the manuscript.
O	We have **deleted** the word appended.
E	The most frequently used word in this context is **deleted**. **Erased** is wrong. The word **removed** can also be used, but is less frequent.

✗	The manuscript is not **adapted to** the journal guidelines.
O	The manuscript does not **follow** the journal guidelines.
O	The manuscript does not **meet** the journal guidelines.
O	The manuscript does not **match** the journal guidelines.
O	The manuscript does not **adhere to** the journal guidelines.
E	In this case, the word **adapted** is incorrect. Adapted means modified or changed. The word **follow** is better. It would also be possible to use, **meet**, **match**, **adhere to** the journal guidelines.

X	**Please understand** that values come from a wide range of locations.
O	**We would like to stress** that values come from a wide range of locations.
O	**We would like to emphasize** that values come from a wide range of locations.
O	**We would like to point out that** values come from a wide range of locations.
E	The expression '**please understand**' cannot be used in this situation. Possible expressions are as follows: **We would like to stress/emphasize/point out that** values come from a wide range of locations.

X	This information was **missed** in the original manuscript.
O	This information was **missing** in the original manuscript.
O	This information was **not included** in the original manuscript.
O	This information was **not in** the original manuscript.
E	**Missed** in this context is incorrect. The correct pattern is, **X was missing** or **X was not included**.

X	We agree with your suggestions. **Actually**, we are **just** investigating the efficacy of this treatment.
O	We are **currently** investigating the efficacy of this treatment.
E	The sentence **We agree with your suggestions** is redundant. The words **actually** and **just** are too informal. The word **actually** can be deleted and **just** changed to **currently** or **at present**. These changes make the reply shorter and more formal. It would also be possible to omit the word **currently**. The shortest response is, **We are investigating the efficacy of this treatment**.

✗	All background information should be **concentrated to** the Introduction.
○	All background information **should be in** the Introduction.
E	The best expression is **should be in**. The word **concentrated** in this context is unnecessary

✗	The comment from Reviewer 2 is **reasonable**.
○	**We agree with** the comment made by reviewer 2 concerning (topic).
○	**We accept the point** made by reviewer 2 concerning (topic).
○	**We take the point** concerning (topic).
E	In this case, the most commonly used expressions are **agree with the point/comment**, **accept the point**, and **take the point**. It is not usual to refer to reviewers' comments as **reasonable**. The shortest response is as follows: **We take the point concerning X**.

✗	In response to this **notice**, we revised the sentence as follows: (show revised sentence)
○	In response to this **comment**, we revised the sentence as follows: (show revised sentence)
○	**We revised the sentence as follows:** (show revised sentence).
E	The word **notice** is incorrect and should be changed to **comment**.

✗	We **appreciate** the reviewers for their useful comments.
○	We **thank** the reviewers for their useful comments.
○	**We appreciate the reviewers' comments.**
○	**We appreciate the useful comments from the reviewers.**
○	**We appreciate the reviewers' helpful comments and suggestions.**
○	**Thank you for your comments.**
E	The expression **We appreciate the reviewers for their useful comments** is incorrect. It is, however, possible to say **We appreciate the useful comments from the reviewers. We appreciate the reviewer's helpful comments and suggestions.**
✗	We have added several sentences **for stress** the importance of the choice of locations.
○	We have added several sentences **to stress/stressing** the importance of the choice of locations.
○	**To stress the importance of** the choice of locations, we have added several sentences.
○	**To emphasize the importance of** the choice of locations, we have added several sentences.
E	In this case, the correct grammar is **to stress** or **stressing**. In the second example, the word **stress** comes at the beginning of the sentence in the phrase, **to stress the importance of X**. The word **emphasize** can also be used.

✗	**We did not perform this time a study of** young people.
○	**We did not focus on** young people in this study.
○	**We did not look at** young people in this study.
○	Young people **were not the focus of this study**.
○	Young people **were excluded from this study**.
E	The word **perform** is usually used as follows: **to perform an experiment**. The easiest way to express this situation is with the two-word verb **focus on**. Another possible verb is **look at**. For example, **We did not focus on/look at young people in this study**. **Focus** can be used as a noun as in the third example. Young people **were not the focus of this study**.

✗	Thank you for **mentioning** this error.
○	Thank you for **pointing out** this error.
○	Thank you for **bringing this error to our attention**.
E	While it is possible to use the word mention, it is better to use more formal verbs such as **point out** or **bring X to our attention**. In addition to the word error, you can use **point**, **problem** or **issue**.

✗	To explain **above** reactions, we have added the following equations.
○	To explain **the above reactions**, we have added the following equations.
E	Before the word **above**, it is necessary to have **the**. The correct usage is as follows: **the above reactions**, **the above discussion**, **the above equation**, **the above data** and so on. However, the following sentence is possible. **This data is shown above**. In this case, an article is not necessary before the word above.

✗	We greatly **appreciated** the **fruitful** comments. We would like to express our **heartfelt** thanks.
○	**Thank you for your useful comments**.
○	**Thank you for your helpful comments and suggestions**.
E	The main problem with this response is that the words **appreciate**, **fruitful** and **heartfelt** are too formal to use in responses to reviewers comments. In this situation, a short and simple sentence such as **Thank you for your useful comments** is sufficient.
✗	The title has been **modified to** Prevention and treatment of dental caries.
○	The title has been **changed to** 'Prevention and treatment of dental caries'.
○	The title has been **changed as follows:** 'Prevention and treatment of dental caries'.
○	**The revised title is as follows:** (show revised title).
○	**We have modified the title, which now reads as follows:** (show revised title)
○	**The title has been modified as follows:** 'Prevention and treatment of dental caries'.
E	The word modified cannot be followed by 'to'. **Modified** refers to very small, minor changes. **Changed** is more frequently used. The last two examples show how to correctly use the word **modified**. The shortest response is, **The revised title is as follows:** (show revised title).

3. Expressions

✗	Changes to the manuscript are shown **in red letters**.
○	Changes to the manuscript are **shown in red**.
○	Changes to the manuscript are **in red**.
E	The correct expression is **shown in red** or **in red**. The words **letters** or **characters** are not necessary.

✗	**We regret to say** we could not obtain that data.
○	**Unfortunately,** we could not obtain that data.
○	**We were unable to** obtain that data.
○	**That data was unobtainable**.
E	The expression **we regret to say** is too formal and has been changed to **unfortunately**. The best response is the shortest. **That data was unobtainable**.

✗	**Thank you for your review and consideration of our manuscript while you are very busy**.
○	**Thank you for your useful comments**.
○	**Thank you for reviewing our manuscript**.
E	The expression **while you are very busy** is a direct translation from Japanese and cannot be used in English in this situation.

✗	This sentence has been **revised to** 'Particles were stored in a sterile environment'.
○	This sentence has been **revised as follows:** 'Particles were stored in a sterile environment'.
○	**We have revised this sentence as follows:** 'Particles were stored in a sterile environment'.
○	**The revised sentence now reads as follows:** 'Particles were stored in a sterile environment'.
○	**This sentence has been changed to** 'Particles were stored in a sterile environment'.
E	The expression **has been revised as follows** is commonly used. However, **changed to** is possible. For example, **This sentence has been changed to** 'Particles were stored in a sterile environment'.

✗	**Sorry for the Conclusion**. The last two sentences have been deleted.
○	**We apologize for** the mistake in the Conclusion. The last two sentences have been deleted.
○	**We have deleted the last two sentences of the Conclusion**.
E	The expression **sorry for the conclusion** is too informal. An apology is unnecessary and has been omitted from example 2.

✗	This sentence has been changed to **the suggested sentence**.
○	We have changed the sentence **as suggested**.
○	We have adopted **the suggested sentence**.
○	**We have adopted the sentence suggested by the reviewer**.
E	The original sentence is too wordy because **sentence** appears twice. Please note that the word **adopted** in examples 2 and 3 means **accepted** or **chosen**. Care should be taken not to confuse the words **adopted** and **adapted**. 'Adapted' means **changed** or **modified**.

✗	The comments and suggestions <u>are very valuable to improve the scientific impact of our manuscript</u>.
○	**We feel that our manuscript has improved considerably as a result of the input received from the editor and the reviewers.**
○	**The comments received from the editor and reviewers have helped us to improve the manuscript.**
E	It is not necessary to comment in detail on particular aspects of the paper that have been improved as a result of the reviewers' comments. Your responses should be as short, detached and formal as possible.

✗	<u>As you suggested,</u> we have improved the quality of Figure 2.
○	**The quality of Figure 2 has been improved.**
○	**We have improved the quality of Figure 2.**
○	**We have changed/modified Figure 2 to make it easier to understand.**
E	It is not necessary to use the phrase **as you suggested** at the beginning of every response to a reviewer's comment. Using the passive form **has been improved** is more formal and detached than **we have improved**, but both are possible. The shortest response is as follows: **Figure 2 has been revised.**

✗	<u>As you kindly suggested,</u> we have included all of the statistical results.
○	**We have included all of the statistical results.**
○	**We included all of the statistical results.**
○	**All of the statistical results have been included.**
E	The phrase, **as you kindly suggested**, is redundant and can be deleted. In general, excessive use of '**As you suggested**' and '**As suggested by the reviewer**' should be avoided.

✗	<u>I tried to accommodate each item</u> that has been pointed out by the reviewers.
○	**We have addressed all of the points** made by the reviewers.
○	**We have addressed all the issues** raised by the reviewers.
○	**We have dealt with the points** raised by the referees as follows.
E	The word **addressed** is more appropriate than **accommodate**. **Deal with** is also possible. Rather than **item**, a better word is **points**. The word **issues** can also be used.
✗	<u>I show correspondence for</u> the comments as follows.
○	**Please find below detailed responses to the reviewers' comments**.
E	The expression **I show correspondence for the comments as follows** is incorrect. Please note that the example sentence given here comes just below the opening paragraph of your responses to reviewers and before the detailed list of responses. The word **below** refers to the list of responses to comments.
✗	We rewrote the description to emphasize the main points and <u>add the implications</u>.
○	We rewrote the description to emphasize the main points and **explain the implications**.
E	The word **implications** is usually preceded by the word **explain** in the phrase **to explain the implications**.

✗	We greatly appreciate the **positive tone** in your review of our manuscript and your **invaluable advice**.
○	**Thank you for your useful comments and suggestions, which we greatly appreciate.**
○	**Thank you for your useful comments and suggestions.**
E	The expression **the positive tone** is not appropriate because it suggests that the author is judging the reviewer's comments. The phrase **invaluable advice** is an exaggeration and should be avoided. Better expressions are as follows: **useful advice**, **helpful advice**.
✗	**We were very sorry for this mistake**. The locations used were all in southeast England and no locations outside the UK were used in this study.
○	In the original manuscript, **we incorrectly stated that** locations outside the UK were used. This description has been deleted. **We apologize for this mistake**.
E	The sentence **we were very sorry** should be in the present tense. To increase the formality, I have changed it to **We apologize for this mistake**. In general, **it is not necessary to apologize** when responding to a reviewer's comment, and expressions such as **we are very sorry** should be avoided. When referring to an error, a useful phrase is **we incorrectly stated that**, **it was incorrectly stated that**.
✗	We revised the sentence **along with** your comments.
○	We revised the sentence **in line with** your comments.
○	We revised the sentence **based on** your comments.
○	We revised the sentence **in accordance with** your comments.
E	The expression **along with** is incorrect because it means **together with**. It should be changed to **in line with**, which means **according to**. It is also possible to use the phrase **based on**. The shortest response is as follows: **This sentence has been revised**.

✗	Another reviewer **was claimed this point**.
○	**The same issue has been raised** by another reviewer.
○	**The same point** was made by another reviewer.
○	Another reviewer **made the same point**.
○	Another reviewer **made the same criticism**.
E	The grammar **X was claimed** is incorrect. It is better to start with, **The same issue**, **The same point**. Another way to say the same thing is with the expression **to raise an issue**. **The same issue has been raised by reviewer two**. **Another reviewer raised the same issue**.

✗	We **deeply appreciate** all the comments made by the reviewers.
○	**Thank you for your comments and suggestions**.
E	The expression **deeply appreciate** is too formal. A more neutral and natural expression is **Thank you for your useful comments and suggestions**.

✗	Thank you very much for your **kind suggestions for our study**.
○	**Thank you for your comments**.
E	The sentence, **thank you very much for your kind suggestions for our study**, is unnecessary and has no meaning. It should not be used excessively in responses to reviewers' comments.

✗	**I am grateful I got appropriate** comments from the reviewers.
○	**I would like to thank the reviewers for their helpful comments and suggestions**.
○	**Thank you for your useful comments and suggestions**.
E	The expression, **I am grateful I got appropriate comments**, is not suitable as a response to a reviewer. In particular, the word **appropriate** is a problem because it suggests the author is evaluating the quality of the reviewer's comment.

✗	We added the following sentences to **perspective to the data**.
○	We added the following sentences to **put the data in perspective**.
E	When using the word **perspective**, the most common structure is **to put** (something) **in perspective**.

✗	**These items** are reflected in the revised manuscript.
○	**All of the reviewers' suggested changes have been incorporated in the revised manuscript**.
○	**All of the reviewers' suggested changes have been included in the revised manuscript**.
○	**All of the reviewers' suggested changes are reflected in the revised manuscript**.
E	Instead of **these items**, a better expression is **all of the reviewers' suggested changes**.

✗	We changed the explanation in **a way suggested by the reviewer**.
○	We changed the explanation **in line with the reviewer's comment**.
○	We changed the explanation **based on the reviewer's comment**.
E	The expression **in a way suggested by the reviewer** is incorrect. **In line with** is more frequently used. **Based on** is also possible.

Part 7
Index of frequently used words

Listed below you will find examples of frequently used words in responses to reviewers' comments. The words are arranged in alphabetical order and examples given.

A

Account — We have **taken into account** the reviewers' comments and revised the manuscript accordingly.

According to — We have formatted the references **according to** the Author Guidelines.

Add — The percentage increase **has been added to** Figure 1.

Addition — **In addition**, the Figure legends have been checked and revised where necessary.

Additional — We have conducted **additional** experiments. Analysis of the data is included on page 7.

Address — We have **addressed** the grammar and syntax problems pointed out by the reviewer.

Agree — We **agree** that the term handicapped is unacceptable. It has been changed to physically challenged.

Appropriate — We believe that our manuscript is **appropriate** for publication in the Journal of Oral Science.

Attach — Please find **attached** the revised version of our manuscript entitled, 'Lifestyle factors and gum disease'.

Avoid — We have **avoided** using the term handicapped in the revised manuscript as it is now unacceptable.

B

Base on — **Based on** the reviewer's comments, we have thoroughly revised the paper.

C

Change — Figure 2 **has been changed** so that it includes the age and sex of the participants.

Check — We **have checked** the list of references and made corrections to references 12, 15 and 19. (show the corrected references)

Cite — We **have cited** three references to support the information on page 6.

Clarify	To **clarify** this point, we have rewritten the sentences as follows: (show revised version)
Clarity	This section has been revised for **clarity** and now reads as follows: (show revised version)
Comment	Thank you for your **comment** concerning onset of the disease. We have revised this sentence.
Comments	Thank you for your useful **comments** and suggestions.
Correct	The grammar errors **have been corrected** by a native speaker of English.

D

Deal with	We **have dealt with** the issues raised by the reviewers as follows: (show list of responses)
Delete	The term physically handicapped **has been deleted** from the manuscript.
Demonstrate	As previous studies **have demonstrated**, the system can be stabilized by the addition of more adhesive.
Describe	The main differences between the modified apparatus and the standard one **have been described** in the second paragraph on page 7 of the revised manuscript.
Detailed	Please find below **detailed** responses to the points raised by the reviewers.
Details	We have provided more **details** of the newly developed technology on page 7, lines 17 - 23.
Determine	The level of concentration was **determined** and the information added to the text.
Disagree	For the following reasons, we **disagree** with the reviewer's comment that 'results are too preliminary to be of interest'. (show a numbered list of reasons)
Discussion	We added several sentences to the **Discussion** concerning the type of land use and factors related to pollution.
Documented	It is **well-documented** that biodegradable polymers have applications in the packaging industry.

Drop············· We have **dropped** the section on biodegradable polymers.

E

Employ············· The measurement methods **employed** have been more fully explained in the Methods section.

Examine············· We hope to **examine** the question of reliability in a future paper.

Explain············· The method employed by Ueda et al. 2015 has been briefly **explained** in the revised manuscript.

F

Find············· Please **find** below our responses to the reviewers' comments.

Follow············· The revised references are as **follows**: (show revised version)

Following············· The **following** sentence has been added to the Discussion section.

G

Grateful············· We are **grateful** to the reviewers for carefully reading our manuscript and providing us with useful advice and comments.

H

Hypothesis············· The **hypothesis** of this study has been added to lines 71-72 of the revised manuscript.

Hypothesize············· We **hypothesized** that location sites selected for antennas were influenced by the proximity of overhead electric cables.

I

Improve············· The quality of the images in Figure 7 **has been improved**.

Include············· We **have included** more data on the experimental setup on page 7, lines 15 – 21 of the revised manuscript.

Incorporate············· All of the reviewers' suggestions **have been incorporated** in the revised manuscript.

Interest	The findings reported here will be **of interest to** readers of the Journal of Oral Science.

L

Line	We have made substantial changes to the Discussion section **in line with** the reviewers' comments.
List	Details of corrections made to the manuscript are **listed** below.

M

Major	The **major** changes we have made are as follows: (show a numbered list of major changes)
Manuscript	The revised **manuscript** is attached.
Mean	This **means** that the system can be applied in a variety of environments.
Meet	We trust that the revised manuscript will **meet** with the approval of the editor and the reviewers.
Misleading	The description on page 8, lines 26 - 30 is **misleading** and has been deleted.
Mistake	As pointed out, there was a **mistake** in the percentage data in Table 4. This has been corrected.
Move	The description concerning degrees of pollution **has been moved** to the Discussion section.

N

Note	The reviewer correctly **notes** that the literature review is missing several key references. We have cited three of the most relevant papers.

O

Omit	We **have omitted** the time-course data in Figures 7 and 9.
Original	In the **original** manuscript, we used the word 'handicapped'. This has been changed to 'physically challenged'.

P

Part — This **part** of the original manuscript has been deleted.

Perform — Experiments **were performed** on days 2, 5 and 7. This information has been added.

Plan — We **plan** to carry out further experiments in the near future.

Point — We **take the reviewer's point** concerning the age of onset, and have included two references that report cases of men in their 20's showing signs of the disease.

The **point** we wanted to make was that the reliability of the system has been improved.

Point out — Thank you for **pointing out** the notation error. It has been changed as follows: (show revised version)

Previously — **Previously**, we reported that degradation was a two-stage process.

Provide — We have **provided** a short paragraph on the possible future applications of the technology described.

Put forward — More information has been added to page 7 to support the hypothesis **put forward** in the Introduction.

Q

Quality — We have improved the **quality** of Figure 2.

Query — The reviewer has **queried** our use of the term physically handicapped. We agree that it is no longer acceptable and have deleted it from the manuscript.

Question — The reviewer has **questioned** our use of external sites. A more detailed description has been added to the text.

Questionable — The reviewer feels that our use of outside sites is **questionable**. A more detailed description has been added to the text.

R

Raise — We have addressed the main issues **raised** by the reviewers.

Read	The revised sentence now **reads** as follows: (show revised version)
Reasons	For the **reasons** given above, we are unable to provide this data.
Rectify	The legends for Figures 4 and 5 are not correct. This problem **has been rectified**.
Refer	Please **refer** to our detailed answer to comment no. 17.
Reference	We agree that the information contained in **reference** 27 is not directly related and have deleted it.
References	We have revised **references** 9, 12 and 17.
Regarding	**Regarding** the possibility that rates of biodegradability may be affected by conditions, we have added several lines to the Discussion section.
Relevant	We think that our manuscript is **relevant** to the scope and aims of the journal.
Remove	We have **removed** the phrase, 'it could be argued' from the manuscript.
Reorganize	The Results section was **reorganized** in response to criticism from both reviewers.
Repetition	We agree that there is too much **repetition** in the Discussion section. We have deleted the description on page 12, lines 17 - 27.
Rephrase	Considering the reviewer's comments, we have **rephrased** the first two lines of the Introduction.
Report	We **report** the results of a study focusing on the connection between denture wearing at night and pneumonia in people over the age of 85.
Response	Please find below our **responses** to the reviewers' comments.
Retain	We wish to **retain** the figure in its present form.
Revise	This section **has been revised** to improve clarity.
Reword	Based on the reviewer's comments, we have **reworded** the title of the paper, which is now as follows: (show revised title)
Rewrite	Page 3, line 7 **has been rewritten** as follows: (show revised version)

S

Say	What we wanted to **say** was that the increase was intermittent.
See	Please **see** our response to comment #17.
Show	Our previous study **showed** that the optimum number of sites was 18.
Should	In reference 12, the year is incorrect. It **should** be 2014.
State	The rate of increase **has been stated** in line 78 of the revised manuscript.
Statement	The following **statement** has been added to the text. (show the added statement)
Submit	I am pleased to **submit** an original article entitled (title) by (names of authors) for consideration for publication in the Journal of Oral Science.
Suggest	We have changed the text as **suggested**.
Suggestion	Thank you for your useful **suggestions**.
Summarize	Important information on site location and sampling techniques **has been summarized** in Table 3.

T

Terms	**In terms of** thermodynamic data, similar rates have been reported by Stuart 2014 and Billison 2015.
Text	Information concerning stability has been added to the **text** on page 5.
Think	We **think** that the poor connection between sites was caused by the choice of location.

U

Unclear	We accept that the Conclusion is **unclear** in places and have revised this section.

V

Validity ·············· We have added some sentences to the text to support the **validity** of the tests employed.

W

Wording ·············· The **wording** of the legends in Figures 7 and 8 has been changed based on the reviewer's comments.

Notes on responding to reviewers' comments

Don't get mad, get formal
査読コメントへの対応は，腹を立てず，丁寧に

Few papers are accepted without the need for revision and most will require major revision. How authors respond to the need for revisions will have a significant impact on the outcome of the submission. Here are some suggestions that I hope will help you.
1. After you have read the reviewers' comments, put them aside for a few days and think about them.
2. If necessary, show the comments to a coworker and ask for advice.
3. Start drafting responses to the comments and taking action where necessary, such as considering extra experiments, adding references and so on.
4. When it comes to writing responses, my advice is as follows: <u>Don't get mad, get formal</u>. What do I mean by this? Well, I mean that it is not wise to let your anger or frustration show in your responses. I also mean that it is better to use formal academic English in your response.

I recently came across a case where the author had been asked to perform an additional experiment. The problem was that the submission deadline for the revised paper was within six weeks. The authors replied in the following way.

- *As the reviewer should know, it is completely impossible to conduct an additional experiment and get reliable data in just six weeks.*

In the above response, the expressions 'as the reviewer should know' and 'it is completely impossible' are too direct and hence somewhat impolite. Below I have rewritten the original response in more formal English and explained each of the main steps.

We note that the reviewer requires further experiments to verify several points made in the manuscript, and that the deadline set for resubmission is six weeks from now. Given the time required to set up and complete the experiments, and analyze the data, we regret to say that we will be unable to meet the deadline.

1. Summarize the reviewer's request
   '*We note that the reviewer requires further experiments to verify several points made in the manuscript,*'
2. State any facts concerning the reviewers' comments
   '*and that the deadline set for resubmission is six weeks from now.*'
3. Give reasons why you cannot meet the request
   '*Given the time required to set up and complete the experiments, and analyze the data, we regret to say that we will be unable to meet the deadline.*'

【著者略歴】
C.S.Langham

1976年　ハダースフィールド大学卒業
1982年　ケント大学大学院修了
2000年　日本大学歯学部教授（英語）
2020年　日本大学特任教授

国際論文 English　投稿ハンドブック
カバーレター作成・査読コメントへの返答　ISBN978-4-263-43361-4

2017年 1 月10日　第 1 版第 1 刷発行
2022年 4 月10日　第 1 版第 3 刷発行

　　　　　　　　　　　　　　　著　者　C. S. Langham
　　　　　　　　　　　　　　　発行者　白 石 泰 夫
　　　　　　　　　　　　　　発行所　医歯薬出版株式会社
　　　　　　　　〒113-8612　東京都文京区本駒込 1 － 7 － 10
　　　　　　　　　　　　TEL.（03）5395-7638（編集）・7630（販売）
　　　　　　　　　　　　FAX.（03）5395-7639（編集）・7633（販売）
　　　　　　　　　　　　　　https://www.ishiyaku.co.jp/
　　　　　　　　　　　　　　郵便振替番号 00190-5-13816

乱丁，落丁の際はお取り替えいたします　　　印刷・あづま堂印刷／製本・愛千製本所
© Ishiyaku Publishers, Inc., 2017. Printed in Japan

本書の複製権・翻訳権・翻案権・上映権・譲渡権・貸与権・公衆送信権（送信可能化権を含む）・口述権は，医歯薬出版（株）が保有します．
本書を無断で複製する行為（コピー，スキャン，デジタルデータ化など）は，「私的使用のための複製」などの著作権法上の限られた例外を除き禁じられています．また私的使用に該当する場合であっても，請負業者等の第三者に依頼し上記の行為を行うことは違法となります．

[JCOPY]＜出版者著作権管理機構 委託出版物＞
本書をコピーやスキャン等により複製される場合は，そのつど事前に出版者著作権管理機構（電話 03-5244-5088, FAX 03-5244-5089, e-mail : info@jcopy.or.jp）の許諾を得てください．

大好評！「国際論文 English」シリーズ

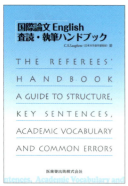

国際論文 English
査読・執筆ハンドブック

C.S.Langham 著

英語論文　査読・執筆　もう怖くない！

◆査読レポートの基本的な構成と書き方を，つづいて査読レポートでよく使われる 200 語について例文を交えながら解説．また，査読レポートを書くなかでおかしやすい単語，文法，言い回しの誤りを，例を挙げて取り上げています．査読レポートを効果的に書くためのアドバイスも掲載．

■ A5判／160頁／2色
■ 定価 3,850 円（本体 3,500 円＋税 10％）ISBN978-4-263-43347-8

姉妹編「国際学会 English」シリーズ！

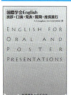

国際学会 English
挨拶・口演・発表・質問・座長進行

C.S.Langham 著
■ B6判／210頁／2色　■ 定価 2,750 円（本体 2,500 円＋税 10％）

国際学会 English
スピーキング・エクササイズ
口演・発表・応答

C.S.Langham 著

音声CD付

■ A5判／120頁／2色　■ 定価 3,300 円（本体 3,000 円＋税 10％）

国際学会 English
ポスター発表

C.S.Langham 著
■ A5判／128頁／2色　■ 定価 3,080 円（本体 2,800 円＋税 10％）

国際学会 English
口頭発表
研究発表のための英語プレゼンテーション

C.S.Langham 著
■ A5判／240頁／2色　■ 定価 3,300 円（本体 3,000 円＋税 10％）

医歯薬出版株式会社

〒113-8612 東京都文京区本駒込1-7-10　TEL.03-5395-7610　FAX.03-5395-7611　https://www.ishiyaku.co.jp/